POSTCARDS from the BUMP

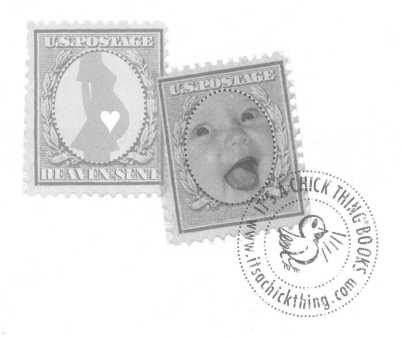

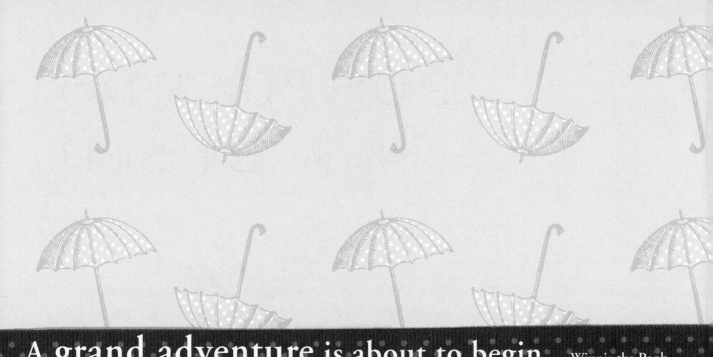

A grand adventure is about to begin. —Winnie the Pooh

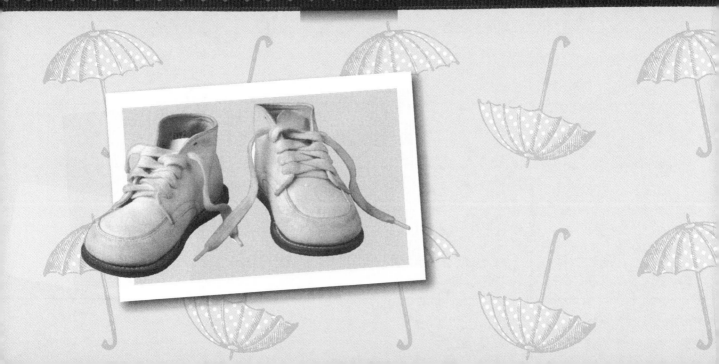

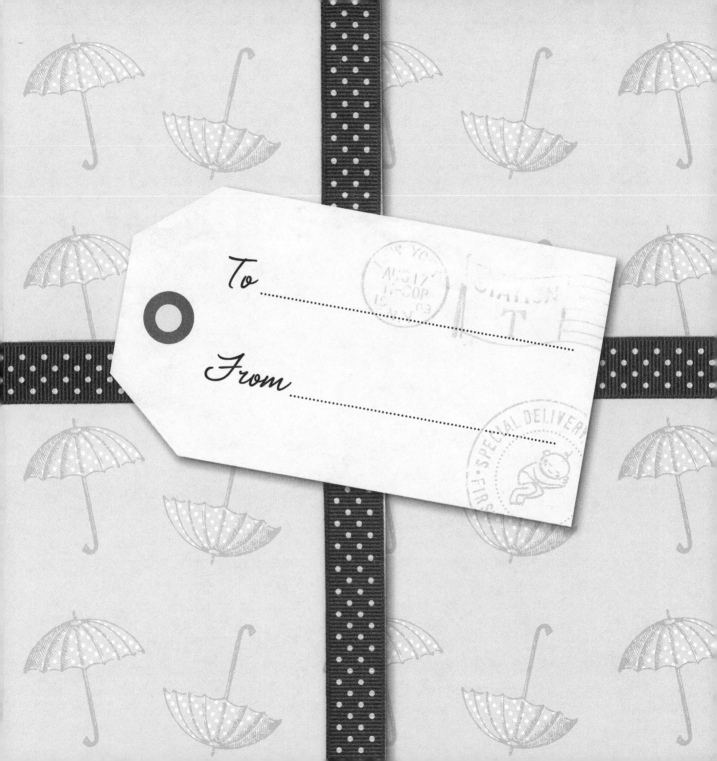

To ....

From ....

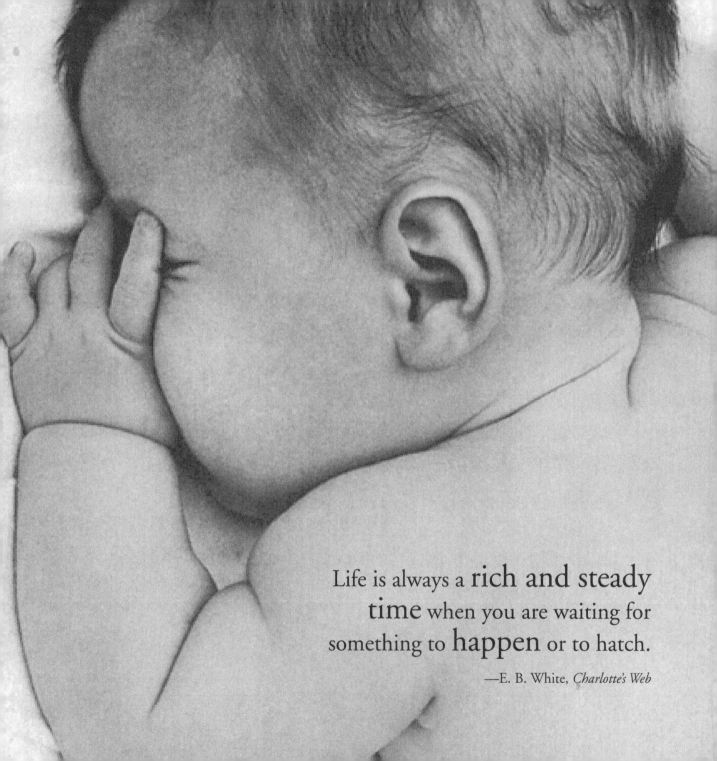

Life is always a **rich and steady time** when you are waiting for something to **happen** or to hatch.

—E. B. White, *Charlotte's Web*

POSTCARDS from the BUMP

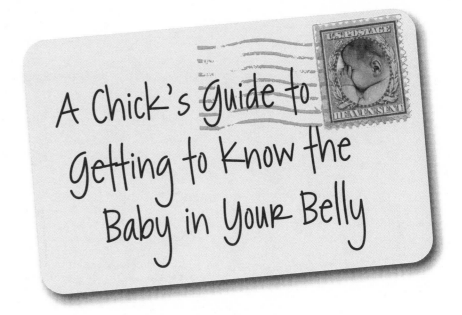

A Chick's Guide to Getting to Know the Baby in Your Belly

U.S. POSTAGE

HEAVEN SENT

AME MAHLER BEANLAND & EMILY MILES TERRY

authors of the *New York Times* Bestseller *Nesting: It's a Chick Thing*®

Copyright © 2009 by Ame Mahler Beanland and Emily Miles Terry
an It's a Chick Thing® book www.itsachickthing.com

Set by the Perseus Books Group

Cataloging-in-Publication data for this book is available from the Library of Congress.

First Da Capo Press edition 2009
ISBN: 978-0-7382-1322-4

Published by Da Capo Press
A Member of the Perseus Books Group
www.dacapopress.com

Note: The information in this book is true and complete to the best of our knowledge. In no way is this book intended to replace, countermand, or conflict with the advice given to you by your own physician. The ultimate decision concerning care should be made between you and your doctor. We strongly recommend you follow his or her advice. Information in this book is general and is offered with no guarantees on the part of the authors or Da Capo Press. The authors and publisher disclaim all liability in connection with the use of this book.

Da Capo Press books are available at special discounts for bulk purchases in the U.S. by corporations, institutions, and other organizations. For more information, please contact the Special Markets Department at the Perseus Books Group, 2300 Chestnut Street, Suite 200, Philadelphia, PA 19103, or call (800) 810-4145, ext. 5000, or e-mail special.markets@perseusbooks.com.

10 9 8 7 6 5 4 3 2 1

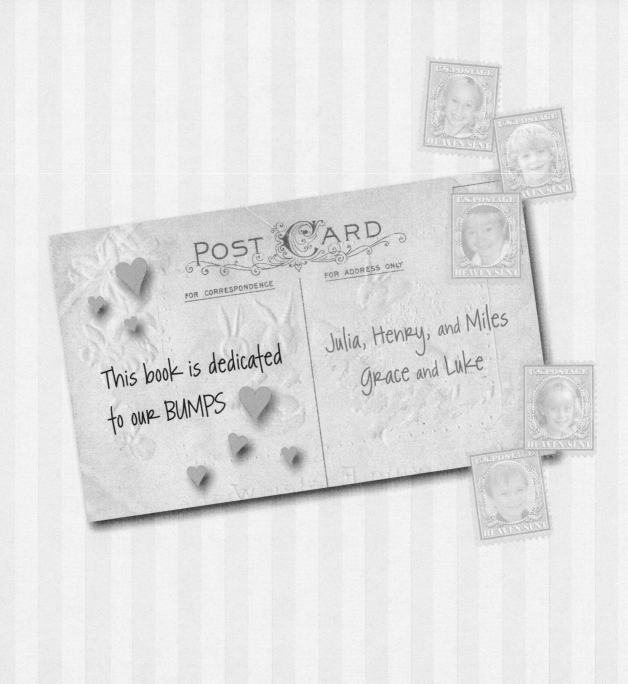

POST CARD

FOR CORRESPONDENCE

FOR ADDRESS ONLY

This book is dedicated to our BUMPS

Julia, Henry, and Miles

Grace and Luke

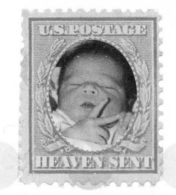

Making the decision

to have a child—

it's momentous. It is

to decide forever to have

your heart go walking around

outside your body.

—Elizabeth Stone

c o n t e n t s

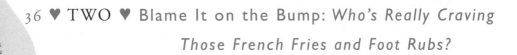

Introduction ❧ What are you waiting for?

Congratulations! You're a mom. . . . Don't be confused—we know you're still sporting a bump and your due date is months, weeks, or days away, but as far as we're concerned, you've already earned the title of "mother." So give yourself a well-deserved pat on the belly. Contrary to popular opinion, we don't see you as a mother-to-be, a pregnant woman, an expectant mother, knocked up, or any of the other terms typically bestowed upon a woman in your shoes. While most of the world insists on treating pregnancy as the waiting period preceding motherhood, we impatiently disagree.

We want to embolden and inspire you to look at your pregnancy in a new and unconventional way—as an opportunity to mother your baby long before he or she is placed in your arms. That bump you are carrying around is not simply a burden to wait out, a bun to bake, a lullaby to practice, or a condition to endure—that's your baby. You don't have to wait for his or her arrival—your little one is already on board, and if you're willing to pay close attention, he or she has a lot to tell you before the birth day rolls around.

Postcards from the Bump is ripe with reasons, inspiration, and solid science to back up the importance of bonding, connecting, and mothering your baby before birth. We've been where you are standing—five times between us—and there are a lot of things we wished we'd known when the maternity shoe was on our foot. While both of us enjoyed reading many of the pregnancy books out there, we felt there was a gap on the bookshelf. We were hungry for a different perspective and had this nagging feeling that many books were holding out on us—as if we could handle only part of the truth. We read countless volumes that provided plenty of helpful information about limb formation, how we should be feeling, what we should eat, and what we needed for baby's nursery. We also read those books that robbed us of precious sleep as we lay awake at night, anxiously certain that we were in the one percent of the population suffering some rare and exotic condition. Instead of wanting to know about what could go wrong or what we needed to buy, we wanted to know about our baby: When and what could our baby hear, feel, and taste? What were our bodies doing to support the baby's development? What was up with all those hormones? Why did this most natural of experiences feel so surreal at times? And mostly, who was this person in my belly?

We wanted the information that would empower us to understand our condition more fully, and we yearned for the permission and encouragement to bond and relate to our babies, long before we were rocking the cradle. So although you may be months away from hearing your baby's first wail or coo, we're going to explain how your baby is already communicating with you via little clues and signals.

"Every pregnancy is different" advise our doctors—and that couldn't be more true.

> Attention
> is the most
> basic form
> of love.
>
> —*John Tarrant*

As any woman who has had more than one child knows, pregnancies are as vastly diverse as the little people they release into the world. With one pregnancy we might crave jalapeno poppers, while with the next we can barely stomach a saltine. With one pregnancy we might look like we've strapped a beach ball to our bellies; the next we might *look* like a beach ball. Some pregnancies are punctuated by bursts of creative energy and drive, while others are mellow experiences in surrender.

I can hear for Miles Shortly after our third child Miles was born I noticed in the hospital how comfortable he was in the arms of his father, sister, and brother, yet when a nurse held him, he'd scream. When we returned home from the hospital, my mother remarked how nice it was that our dog's barking didn't seem to disturb him, and without thinking I said, "Well, he's heard Willie's barking before." And then I realized that that was also why he was so comfortable with family members whose voices he had heard. He already knew a lot about his world, and I found the desire to look back at all the clues Miles had given me as to what he was like. What did I already know about him before he was born? The list was much longer than I could have ever imagined. —*Emily*

We understand that pregnancy is an all-consuming experience, and our goal is to help you nurture both your pre-mom and new-mom personas. We'll give you ideas for ways to pamper yourself—and sound reasons why you should do so—offer creative ways to celebrate your pregnancy milestones, and give you the lowdown on what you'll face when things *really* start to rock.

Above all we believe that if you pay attention to those kicks and turns, hiccups, and more, you'll get a fresh perspective on what it means to be pregnant and a new understanding of that little guy or gal inside.

This book brims with the voices of the many mothers who generously told us about the "postcards" they received from their bumps. Women who were just as nervous about becoming a parent as you might be. Women who figured out through hard-won knowledge, mother's intuition, or gut instinct how to embrace, and not just endure, their pregnancies. And along with rich food for thought, we've snuck in some healthy, delicious recipes that should satisfy your expanding belly.

Our hope is that after you close the book's covers, you'll walk away revived and buoyed, feeling more confident and happy about your pregnancy, yourself, and your baby.

—Ame & Emily

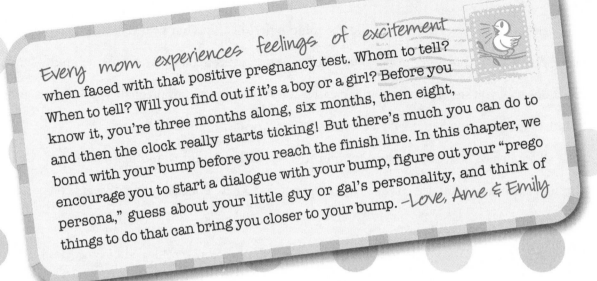

Every mom experiences feelings of excitement when faced with that positive pregnancy test. Whom to tell? When to tell? Will you find out if it's a boy or a girl? Before you know it, you're three months along, six months, then eight, and then the clock really starts ticking! But there's much you can do to bond with your bump before you reach the finish line. In this chapter, we encourage you to start a dialogue with your bump, figure out your "prego persona," guess about your little guy or gal's personality, and think of things to do that can bring you closer to your bump. —Love, Ame & Emily

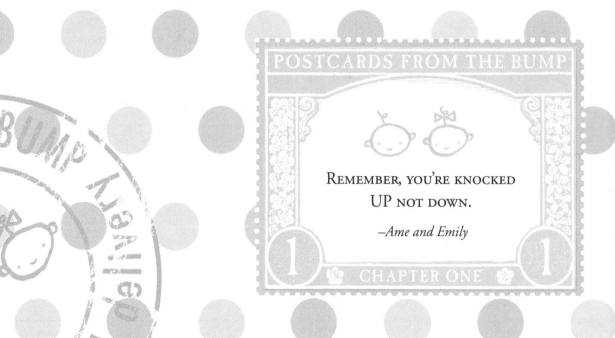

POSTCARDS FROM THE BUMP

REMEMBER, YOU'RE KNOCKED
UP NOT DOWN.

—Ame and Emily

1 · CHAPTER ONE · 1

You've Got Male (or Female)

It's Positive!

Mama's Got a Secret!

Steely reserve is not my hallmark. One margarita is never enough; I'd forgo groceries to buy shoes, and love at first sight? I'm a believer with the wedding ring to prove it. He walked into the room, and I said to my roommate, "There's *my* husband."

Eighteen months later we walked down the aisle. First came love, second came marriage, and when a plus sign heralded our need for a baby carriage, no one was more surprised than I was at my sudden surge of reserve. My husband was astounded when I didn't begin dialing my cell phone from the bathroom with the pregnancy test still in hand.

Before my own pregnancy, I had casually observed the "telling" policies of other women. I knew a large camp of "waiters," who delayed sharing their news until after the first trimester for reasons ranging from superstition and protectiveness to practicality and privacy. I marveled at their tenacity.

I also knew lots of "tellers." Women who dove into the mommy pool head-first—struggling to keep maternity jeans up at five weeks, furnishing lavish nurseries months before due dates, eating double ice-cream sundaes before dinner—and I loved them for it. How could such unchecked optimism be anything but inspiring?

With the maternity shoe firmly on the other foot, though, I found myself squarely camped between the "waiters" and the "tellers." I had always fancied myself a teller, but the reality of pregnancy had me considering defection.

"Let's wait until I've seen the doctor," had been my excuse for waiting to share the happy news with the rest of our family. But when the day finally arrived confirming the most beautiful sound a woman can ever make—a baby's heartbeat—I remained hesitant.

When my husband asked, "Can we tell now?" I was overcome and negotiated for even more time to harbor our sweet secret.

"Can we wait twelve weeks?" I asked, feeling like a complete killjoy.

I was seven weeks pregnant when my thirtieth birthday rolled around. When friends insisted on margaritas, I secretly sipped virgins, while Daddy-to-be covertly shot down the poppers the bartender served me. The day after, my husband was awfully productive for someone who had drunk for two the night before. Up early, he was cooking eggs and bacon when the doorbell rang. Saying that he couldn't leave the stove, he forced me to abandon my cozy perch on the sofa to answer the door. Imagine my shock when I opened it to find my sister, who had been full of apologies for being out of town on my birthday, and my mom, who lived 3,000 miles away.

"Surprise! Happy birthday," he said, grinning.

When he started making "let's tell them" eyes, I balked briefly before it hit me—I couldn't *not* tell my mother and sister the great news in person. And so I ended this pregnant pause in our lives and let my carefully considered resolve to wait 12 weeks fall short by five.

What are you going to do? Life is full of surprises—big ones, little ones, cleverly orchestrated ones, and totally spontaneous ones. And the world is full of mysteries that science can only attempt to explain—sperm permeating egg; positive results activated by hormones; babies under skin one moment, in our arms the next. And with mystery comes fear but also the potential for extraordinary faith and grace. Grace, that's what we named our daughter. An apt name for the little person who continues to teach me that life is indeed all about timing—eating before the ice cream melts, dancing when you hear your favorite song, and never missing the opportunity to hold someone's hand.

I do not at all understand the mystery of grace— only that it meets us where we are but does not leave us where it found us.

—*Anne Lamott*

Postcard *to the* Bump

The first person I told about you was ....
....
....
....
....
....
....
....

People forget to mention how this mysterious little person will **keep you company** every hour of every day, banishing every notion of loneliness for the unforeseeable future, how even though you've yet to meet, you'll **love your growing baby with a ferocity** that makes Superwoman look wimpy, and how glad you'll be that your body knows how to make eyelashes without consulting you.

—*Jennifer Margulis*

Doggone Noisy One day, late into my pregnancy with our second child, Luke, I was sitting on the couch, reading to our four-year-old-daughter, Grace. Luke, who was normally very active, was very still—as if dozing through the story. Suddenly someone knocked at our door and our little dog, Buster, let out this loud bark. I'll never forget the strange feeling of Luke startling in my belly—he literally "jumped" as if jolted from a sound sleep. When I answered the door it was my neighbor Karen, and we laughed about how "she'd woken up the baby." It was one of many "Aha!" moments in my pregnancy that confirmed what I'd felt from the moment I found out I was pregnant—Luke was very present, aware, and hanging out with his family already, and we were just getting to know him from the inside out. To this day Luke loves Buster, but he never fails to jump or be upset when he barks. —Ame

Mommy and Me:
Who's Your Prego Persona?

Whether you're pregnant with your first or you've already got a nest full of baby chicks, you might recognize these mother hens from your maternity store forays or from somewhere much closer to home—as in your very own mirror.

The Gucci Gucci Glamour Mama—

Donning the latest in bump couture from head to toe, she practices artful accessorizing that helps her keep up appearances even as her due date looms and her bump begins to bloom. Sensible flats? Never. This haute mama insists on staying at the height of fashion in high heels. Her secret to keeping it up? Luxurious spa pedicures and frequent foot massages.

The Drama Mama—

She's hot and sweaty and certain it's symptomatic of the rare disorder she just happened to read about in her latest pregnancy book. High maintenance, and always ailing, she keeps her obstetrician's phone line buzzing. Out of prenatal vitamins? Call Drama Mama: She'll adore pulling you into her momtourage and sharing a bottle from her cabinet stocked with formulas that simply didn't agree with her delicate constitution.

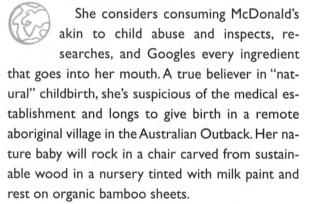

The Earth Mama—

She considers consuming McDonald's akin to child abuse and inspects, researches, and Googles every ingredient that goes into her mouth. A true believer in "natural" childbirth, she's suspicious of the medical establishment and longs to give birth in a remote aboriginal village in the Australian Outback. Her nature baby will rock in a chair carved from sustainable wood in a nursery tinted with milk paint and rest on organic bamboo sheets.

The Muumuu Mama—

She might have started off as a size zero but she quickly blossomed to double digits. No waist? No problem. She loves pushing the boundaries of her maternal ad-

 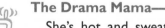

venture and never lets a waistband interfere as she bounces along in voluminous dresses. She insists that she needs milkshakes and Dove Bars daily for the extra calcium and swears French fries are a vegetable.

The Mama-Mia—

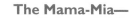

When you say, "Hey baby," she's certain you're talking to her. A veteran of monopolizing conversations, she's ecstatic to have twice as much to share with the world. She's posted her website (with blog), booked her nude pregnancy portrait session and belly mold sculpture appointments months in advance, and has already chosen a tasteful "push present" from Tiffany. Woe to her Baby Daddy who strives to meet her ever-increasing demands for attention, validation, and Philly cheese steaks at 3 a.m.

Alpha-Mom—

This hyperorganized mama chose her baby's nursery colors before she even knew she was knocked up. By her second trimester she's completed her infant care classes, installed the baby's car seat, signed up for daycare, and started researching preschools. Somehow she manages to keep up with her endless to-do list and get to the gym for pregnancy yoga at daybreak.

When your heart speaks, take good notes. —*Judith Campbell*

♥♥ Postcard *to the* Bump ♥♥

When I found out I was expecting you, I felt ....
....
....
....
....
....

Pregnancy is
getting **company**
inside one's skin.

—*Maggie Scarf*

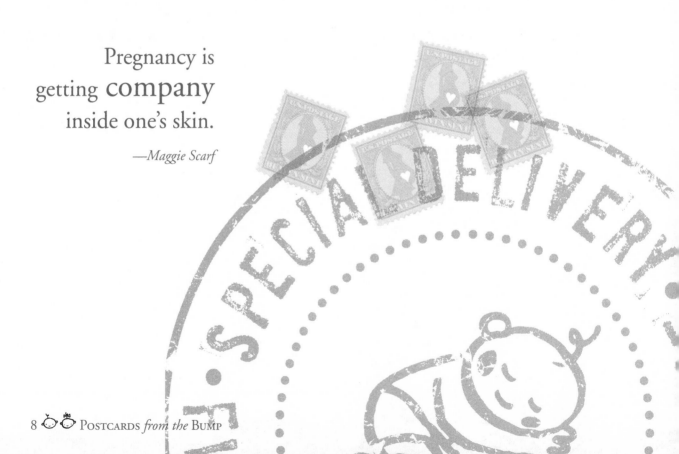

My attitude toward my pregnancy was one of watching an experiment with my uterus. Wasn't this interesting—to see the changes my body was going through! I realize now that I didn't allow myself what I then considered the luxury of excitement and anticipation, though mine was very much a planned and wanted pregnancy. . . . Years later, I learned that babies know what's going on in utero and can hear, feel, and experience emotions long before they're born. When their mothers are detached and not invested emotionally babies sense this.

—*Christiane Northrup, M.D., from* Women's Bodies, Women's Wisdom

Can You Hear Me Now?

Researching prenatal memories is a little tough—while movie stars and babies are equally adept at making grand entrances, babies always flub the red-carpet interview. The studies that do exist, however, suggest compelling evidence that the womb is a baby's first classroom, where learning and memory go hand-in-hand.

One of the most famous studies of newborns, informally dubbed "The Cat in the Hat study," by Drs. Anthony DeCasper and William Fifer, proved that infants recognize their mothers' voices shortly after birth and that this preference is based on prenatal memory. In this study, pregnant women read Dr. Seuss' *The Cat in the Hat* twice a day to their bumps for the last six weeks of their pregnancy. Soon after birth, researchers played a variety of audiotapes to the newborns that corresponded to pacifier-like nipples. After a few trials the little suckers figured out exactly where, and at what rate, to suck in order to tune in to the sound of their mother's voice reading *The Cat in the Hat* as opposed to the recordings of strangers' voices reading another book.

Another group of researchers studied mothers who watched the same soap opera every day throughout their pregnancies. When the theme songs from the programs were played for their newborns, the babies became alert and their heart rates lowered—the same reaction they had when they listened to their mother's voices. Babies who had not "watched the soaps" in utero, however, had no such reaction to the music.

Babies in utero are beginning to learn their native language and can distinguish cadence, rhythm, and intonations. In fact, studies of babies in utero at 26 weeks, have shown that infants already exhibit "speech" behaviors matching their own language, and as soon as they are born they gravitate to the voices of their mother. So, by going about your day chatting as you normally would, you're giving your baby a prenatal language class—that was easy!

Getting to Know You

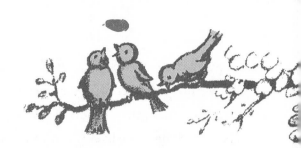

My friend Anne and I wanted our first baby's nurseries to have Pottery Barn rugs, primary colors, and brand-new diaper genies. We both liked baby names that began with *J*. We traded copies of our favorite pregnancy books, with dog-eared alerts to all the scary or funny pages. We nibbled on carrots, avoided fish, and gorged on French fries and milkshakes. Since Anne's due date was a week before mine, she could give me detailed descriptions of all the pregnancy tests ahead of time. "You get to see your whole baby!" she gushed after her 18-week ultrasound, and I relished every word as she told me what to expect. We were pregnant mirrors of each other, blissfully counting down our due dates in unison.

But three weeks before my due date, my pregnant friend jumped ship and abandoned me for, well, motherhood. I vividly remember the afternoon when I listened to the joyful voicemail from Anne's husband—a full ten days ahead of schedule—that said "they had something great to tell us." And then I heard the baby crying in the background. Their beautiful baby boy, Jamie, hadn't been able to wait to get here.

"How'd you do it? How was it?" I peppered her with questions at the hospital just hours after she delivered, and she filled me in. Seeing her cradle her little guy fueled my anticipation, and my pregnant brain decided, in the way that pregnant brains are apt to rashly decide, that our baby would follow suit and come early, too. We visited Jamie several times in the next few days—in the hospital, then later at home. My efforts at putting prenatal peer pressure on my unborn child were in vain, though, as I continued to wait for labor pains. The days crawled by, then came to almost a standstill.

"Have you felt any contractions?" Anne would ask delicately as she nursed.

"Not one," I'd reply.

My due date came and went as Jamie, who was beginning to smile and open his eyes more, seemed to be speeding toward adulthood.

Days ticked by, one week grew into the next, and I couldn't help but ponder the meaning of it all. I wanted to get to know my baby girl so desperately—to see her face, smell her baby breath, cradle her, tickle her. Why was I being cheated out of this extra time with her? Put simply, why was Anne getting more live time with her son than I would with my daughter? When my obstetrician casually informed me that she'd let me go 14 days past my due date before inducing me, something gave way: I realized that to maintain my sanity over the next two weeks, I'd have to forget my due date. My bump was in control.

With newfound resolve, I began to take note of everything I could about my bump. My attention turned from watching the clock to watching my baby. I noticed the times she was awake, her sleepy days, her wakeful days (every other), her hiccups (at least once a day and particularly after I ate something spicy), what she liked to do when I would lie down (flip), or walk (sleep), or when I'd rock in the rocking chair (tap). She bounced and thumped along with the music when I went to a classical music concert. I sat on a bench at the park, patted her, and described to her this place where she might be playing soon. I sat in her nursery and read her *Goodnight Moon*, letting the simple words lull and relax me.

Slowly, I began to feel better. A tenuous peace replaced the anxiousness, and like a mother who finally stops yearning for her child to reach childhood milestones, I stopped wishing the present moment away and learned to enjoy the girl in my belly.

"She has the hiccups again!" I announced to Anne while we watched Jamie squiggle on the floor one day.

"I never noticed that when I was pregnant," she replied.

"You didn't have time to," I laughed.

Now Julia is ten. I tousle her white blonde hair, admire her as she reads for long stretches, tickle her until her cheeks flush pink, and try to remember those moments when I first got to know her by looking deep within my own skin, my own heart, in search of clues to the little person who would enlighten my world.

❀❀ Postcard *to the* Bump ❀❀

When I think about you I feel ....
....
....
....

....
....
....
....
....
....

> We teach our children
> all about life, our
> **children teach us**
> what life is all about.
>
> —*Anonymous*

Making a Date with the Bump

For some pregnant women, feeling connected to our bumps is as easy as shoving a chocolate doughnut in our mouths. For others, it's a struggle to accept that we're actually going to *have a baby*, and we take our own sweet time making the mental leap to motherhood. To help you find your mommy mojo and to learn to enjoy pregnancy a whole lot more, we've found that it helps to spend a little quality time with that bump of yours. Making a "date with your bump" might sound silly, but think of it as whistling while you work—it can make the passage of time and pregnancy a whole lot sweeter. Here are some ideas from other chicks about activities and experiences they enjoyed with their bumps:

TAKE THE BUMP OUT TO PLAY. Soon, you and your baby will be making regular visits together, and a little park/playground tutorial will give you a head start. Begin checking out the local parks in your neighborhood. Online mommy message boards and your city parks and recreation office are great places to scope out what your area has to offer for little ones. Sit on a bench for a while so you can absorb the sights, sounds, and social scene (avoid late afternoons, or the cranky toddlers might send you fleeing and you'll never return!).

BUMP UP THE VOLUME. Whether you like the Ramones or Rachmaninoff, make it a point at some time during your pregnancy to hear some live music. At about six months (and some studies indicate even earlier, around 16 weeks) into your pregnancy, your baby can hear noises from outside the womb, and you may even notice his or her response to the music. Attending a concert hall with great acoustics is equivalent to giving your bump a front-row seat.

BELLY LAUGH. Scientists have found that simply anticipating laughter boosts health-protecting hormones. So whether it's a slapstick movie, a stand-up comic, or a *Seinfeld* rerun, regularly seek out activities that hit your funny bone and get you giggling to give your bump a preview of the good life.

MOMMY AND ME CLASSES. Your baby's brain is growing by leaps and bounds, so why not stretch yours a little, too? Learn something new together. Go to a pregnancy yoga class, learn to knit, take up sudoku puzzles, or learn baby sign language and build some new synapses in your brain.

BOB ALONG, TAKE A DIP. Nothing makes large, bloated bodies feel small again like a swim. Invest in a flattering and comfortable pregnancy bathing suit that will grow along with you, and try to get to a pool regularly. Not only is it relaxing, this low impact exercise will cool your rising temperature and give you and your baby a gravity-defying experience.

The child supplies the power, but the parents have to do the steering.

—*Benjamin Spock*

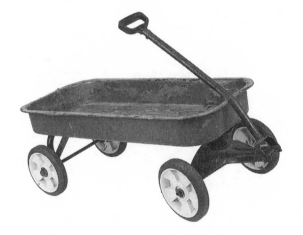

⚭⚭ Postcard *to the* Bump ⚭⚭

One of my favorite places to take you as a bump was ....
....
....
....
....

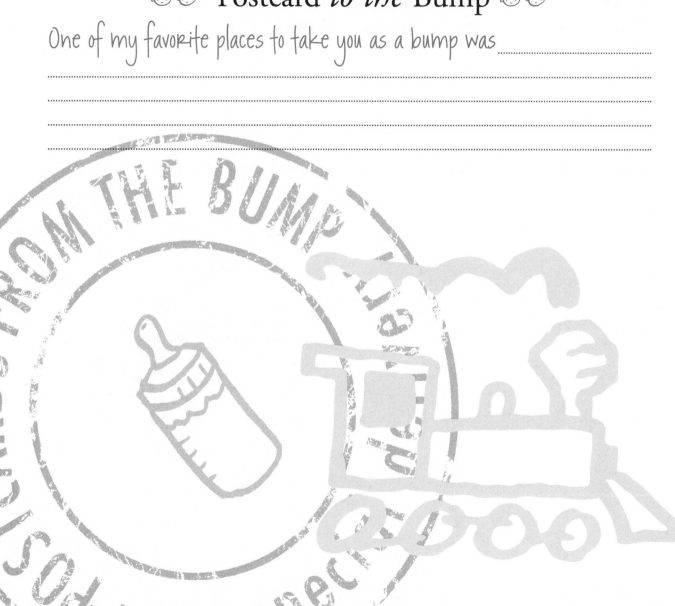

THE BABYMOON: A LITTLE GETAWAY BEFORE LABOR DAY

Falling securely in the pregnancy-just-keeps-getting-better category is the much welcomed "babymoon" tradition. These prenatal getaways for Mom and Dad are designed to give you one last fling before junior (a.k.a., that cute little ball and chain) puts you under house arrest. We highly recommend that you partake in this burgeoning new pregnancy tradition. Typically taken between week 18 and week 24, babymoons come in several different categories:

SOOTHING. For those of us who feel as if our pregnancy experience has hardly been a walk in the park up until now, try a dose of super-concentrated TLC and nonstop pampering. What you need is a trip to a luxurious resort and spa that features prenatal massages, foot rubs, and pools where you can enjoy a swim. Some spas even offer babymoon packages with special prenatal treatments and select activities for the daddy-to-be.

MINDFUL. For the parents-to-be who have a thirst for cultural experiences and feel a drought coming on, now's your chance to play it smart. In other words, unless your baby sleeps 24/7, the only museum in your immediate future is one filled with interactive water displays and throngs of screaming kiddos. Plan a trip to an urban destination with thought-provoking lectures, interesting museums, and cultural sites that will satiate your intellect so you don't feel too put upon when your only semiartistic endeavor becomes your nightly read of *Harold and the Purple Crayon.*

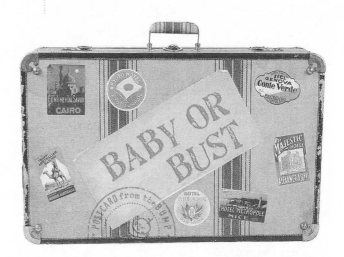

Spirited. Though you might feel like a prego Isaak Denison with a yearn to safari (you even managed to pick up a pink pith helmet and accompanying hat box), the closest you'll get to a live lion now is at your local zoo. Instead, plan a trip to a visually stunning mountainous or coastal region that offers gentle hiking trails, fishing, and canoeing.

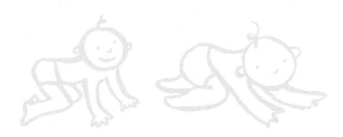

For your bump on the road, you'll want to keep the following in mind:

• Carry a cravings tote: Fill a bag with some of your favorite pregnancy snacks—nutrition bars, nuts, dried fruit, dark chocolate, crackers, and a generously sized water bottle.

• Bring several pairs of ultra-comfortable shoes.

• Pack clothes that enable you to layer so that you can "peel" when you heat up.

• Memorize some recipes of your favorite nonalcoholic drinks so you can instruct bartenders on the road (see p. 75)

• Bring a copy of your medical records.

• Know your blood type.

• If flying, reserve an aisle seat so you can get to the restroom and walk around more easily.

• Avoid mosquitoes and countries with malaria and other health concerns (for more information visit *www.cdc.gov*); if you're hiking, bring bug repellant that will keep ticks away as well.

Sex on the Beach

We had such a BORING ultrasound physician, and when we realized that this expressionless robotron was going to "reveal" our baby's gender, we intervened just in time to ask him to write the gender on our pictures and seal them up in an envelope that we'd take with us. Not long afterward we flew to Kauai for a babymoon vacation. The first morning, I slept in and when I awoke I discovered that my husband had left a note saying, "Bring the ultrasound pictures down to the beach." I did just that, and as we sat watching the waves crash, we decided we'd ask a couple to look in the envelope and write the sex of our baby in the sand. We looked around and found a sweet couple who was willing to "play" our game. They wrote it in the sand, but when David and I turned around, we were puzzled as we tried to figure out what they'd written. We were looking for "boy" or "girl" and our serious, unimaginative doctor had written FEMALE! The couple decoded it for us, and we rejoiced over our baby girl! Upon arriving back in Dallas our families met us at the airport. They had endured the waiting time while we traveled, and our baby's grandparents were dying to know the gender of their first grandbaby. They burst into cheers as they saw us emerge from the airline exit with beautiful pink leis around our necks—we had sent a message that they would know by the color of the leis we were wearing. —Lisa

There are only two ways to live your life. One is as though nothing is a miracle. The other is as though **everything is a miracle.** —*Albert Einstein*

Grasping at Stars:
Who Will Your Bump Be?

Let's face it, we moms get pretty desperate for information on our baby-to-be, and we'll go to great lengths to eek out any little insights into our little ones—even up through the stratosphere. Why not consult the stars and see what your baby's astrological sign might reveal? Take this with a giant grain of salt and remember that unless you're in the labor and delivery room as you read this, his or her sign isn't guaranteed.

Baby Aries • Ram • March 21 to April 19
THE ENERGIZER BABY: Part baby, part motorized machine, your little one will always be on fast-forward. Be prepared if you're about to birth an Aries, because from the moment they're born their adventure-seeking nature will keep you constantly on your toes.
BEST NURSERY DÉCOR: Aries vibe to bright colors, bold patterns, eye-catching pictures, and toys. Wall murals and large-scale art will thrill her.

FAVORITE TOYS: Stock up on batteries! Rams love toys that make sounds, light up, and play music.
MOST LIKELY TO BE FIRST IN YOUR PLAYGROUP TO: Do just about everything.
LEAST LIKELY TO BE FIRST IN YOUR PLAYGROUP TO: Listen quietly to a story.

Baby Taurus
Bull • April 20 to May 20
CREATURE COMFORT CHILD: These family-oriented babies love the soft and cozy, go at their own speed, and adore animals and food.
BEST NURSERY DÉCOR: Surround your baby bull in soft, plush fabrics with animal themes or traditional patterns like toile, gingham, and stripes.
FAVORITE TOYS: Soft teddy bear, "Farmer Says," a set of plastic animals, play kitchen.
MOST LIKELY TO BE FIRST IN YOUR PLAYGROUP TO: Eat a variety of solid foods.
LEAST LIKELY TO BE FIRST IN YOUR PLAYGROUP TO: Crawl.

Baby Gemini • Twins • May 21 to June 21

THE CHATTERBOX: This little baby is curious, talkative, and inquisitive. You'll need a lot of toys and a full schedule of activities to keep her busy and engaged, as you'll want to avoid boredom at all costs.

BEST NURSERY DÉCOR: Geminis are born with style, so indulge your little one with intricate fabrics that have a theme and tell a story or use bold, modern prints to make a unique statement.

FAVORITE TOYS: Play phone, talking toys, "corn popper" push toy.

MOST LIKELY TO BE FIRST IN YOUR PLAYGROUP TO: Speak.

LEAST LIKELY TO BE FIRST IN YOUR PLAYGROUP TO: Listen.

Baby Cancer • Crab • June 22 to July 22

THE CUDDLER: Use your "nice mommy" voice at all times when dealing with this sweetly sensitive babe. Kind, but a bit tearful, your little one needs to feel protected at all times.

BEST NURSERY DÉCOR: To keep Cancers from getting crabby, they need a peaceful, serene retreat. Soft, muted colors, nature-inspired, or traditional themes and clean lines are sure to bring her out of her shell.

FAVORITE TOYS: Soft scrapbook with pictures of their family, plush lamb, or an oft-read book.

MOST LIKELY TO BE FIRST IN YOUR PLAYGROUP TO: Run and cry to their mommy.

LEAST LIKELY TO BE FIRST IN YOUR PLAYGROUP TO: Take a toy from another child.

Baby Leo • Lion • July 23 to August 22

THE KING OR QUEEN OF THE PLAYGROUND: Catch up on your zzzz's before this baby roars onto the scene, because you're about to join the ranks of the massively sleep deprived as your lion's nonstop need for attention will keep you in high gear.

BEST NURSERY DÉCOR: Think royalty for your little lion's den—lush colors, elegant flourishes, mirrors, and sparkle. Be sure to include a big, cozy "throne" for curling up to read and cuddle.

FAVORITE TOYS: A crib mirror, superstar sing-along stage, dress-up clothes, and accessories.

Most likely to be first in your playgroup to: Perform a song-and-dance routine.

Least likely to be the first in your playgroup to: Share.

Baby Virgo • The Virgin • August 23 to September 22

Mommy's Little Helper: Start organizing your house in your first trimester, because this little perfectionist can get fussy if things aren't in order. Happy in his own skin, this little baby likes to help Mommy and Daddy and is always busy in body and mind.

Best Nursery Décor: Little Virgos crave order and tidiness, so decorate their space with sensible geometric patterns and invest in organizing systems to streamline the toys, books, and puzzles in their room.

Favorite Toys: Simple retro-inspired toys, nesting boxes, wooden puzzles, and shape sorters.

Most likely to be the first in your playgroup to: Help clean up toys.

Least likely to be first in your playgroup to: Walk.

Baby Libra • Scales • September 23 to October 22

The Charmer: This little baby might be smiling before you even leave the hospital. Winsome, social, and musical, baby Libras appreciate artistic surroundings.

Best Nursery Décor: Forgo Winnie-the-Pooh and go for more sophisticated and artistic prints and patterns. Libras will especially love a blue or cloud-painted ceiling.

Favorite Toys: Dress-up dolls, Legos, Duplos blocks, easel and paint, and baby instruments.

Most likely to be the first in your playgroup to: Settle a dispute between other babies.

Least likely to be the first in your playgroup to: Appreciate a spooky story.

Baby Scorpio • Scorpio • October 23 to November 21

THE MYSTIFIER: Your baby will long to be the center of attention, yet the reason for her wailing tantrums will be unclear until you really get to know her magnetic and powerful personality.

BEST NURSERY DÉCOR: Scorpios will feel right at home with a canopy over a luxurious crib and a cozy, private nook where they can retreat. Don't be afraid to use deep and jewel-tone colors.

FAVORITE TOYS: Mozart magic music cube, play tent, and dress-up costumes.

MOST LIKELY TO BE THE FIRST IN YOUR PLAYGROUP TO: Successfully complete toilet training.

LEAST LIKELY TO BE THE FIRST IN YOUR PLAYGROUP TO: Graciously take turns.

Baby Sagittarius • The Archer • November 22 to December 21

BORN TO BE WILD: Your baby will be so carefree and happy that other moms will be green with envy. Stay in good shape, because soon you'll be chasing your Sag tike around and around the playground.

BEST NURSERY DÉCOR: Put your little Bohemian at ease in a room that evokes freedom and creativity like ones with wild west, jungle, or fairy themes. Mix old and new for an eclectic, collected-over-time feel for this little one's room.

FAVORITE TOYS: Kite, ball, or ride-on car.

MOST LIKELY TO BE THE FIRST IN YOUR PLAYGROUP TO: Run.

LEAST LIKELY TO BE THE FIRST IN YOUR PLAYGROUP TO: Sit quietly at a coffee shop.

Baby Capricorn • The Goat • December 22 to January 19

THE PLANNER: Your baby will be serious, diligent, and above all, determined. Self-effacing by nature; you will need to toot your baby's horn to get him the credit and attention he deserves.

BEST NURSERY DÉCOR: Corral your little goat in earthy colors, and use natural elements like wood, wicker, and cotton. Be sure to accent his space with maps, quotes, and a generous bookcase.

FAVORITE TOYS: Books, stacking blocks, and coloring books.

MOST LIKELY TO BE THE FIRST IN YOUR PLAYGROUP TO: Speak in full sentences.

MOST LIKELY TO BE THE LAST IN YOUR PLAYGROUP TO: Be toilet trained.

Baby Aquarius • Water Bearer • January 20 to February 18

REBEL BABY: Your baby will be creative, solitary, thoughtful, and bright. You might need to coax out her social side, but rest-assured it's there, and her unique way of looking at things will get her attention wherever she goes.

BEST NURSERY DÉCOR: Think outside the box to create this little one's digs. Forgo juvenile norms and don her crib with an artistic quilt and accessorize with modern art to satisfy her appreciation for contemporary style.

FAVORITE TOYS: Waterwheel play table, paints and crayons, shovel and sand.

MOST LIKELY TO BE THE FIRST IN YOUR PLAYGROUP TO: Pick up a long-ignored toy.

LEAST LIKELY TO BE THE FIRST IN YOUR PLAYGROUP TO: Play with other kids.

Baby Pisces • The Fish • February 19 to March 20

THE DREAMER: Your baby will be very emotional, intuitive, and imaginative. Your caring little one will often demonstrate complete selflessness.

BEST NURSERY DÉCOR: Pisces need to let their imaginations run wild. Outfit his nursery with a vast canvas or corkboard featuring his baby photos and add memorabilia throughout the years for an ever-changing art installation. Paint a wainscoting of chalkboard paint so he can scribble and draw to his heart's desire.

FAVORITE TOYS: Dolls and toy figurines he can use to create his own world.

MOST LIKELY TO BE THE FIRST IN YOUR PLAYGROUP TO: Give all his toys to the other kids.

LEAST LIKELY TO BE THE FIRST IN YOUR PLAYGROUP TO: Give up thumb-sucking.

✿✿ Postcard *to the* Bump ✿✿

Your parents' zodiac signs are ....
....
....
....
....

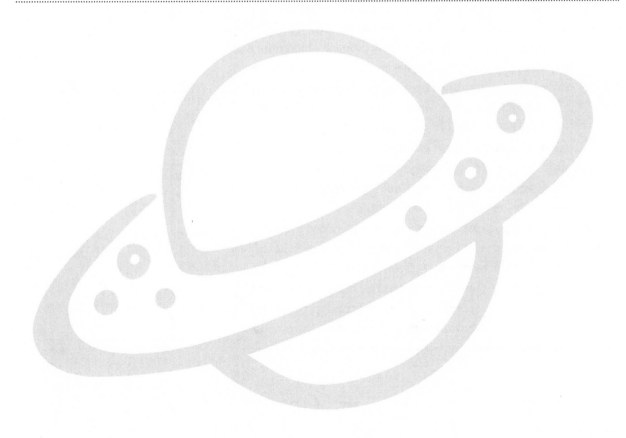

Baby Love

Dubbed the "love" hormone, oxytocin has long been used by doctors to induce labor and increase lactation, but until recently its effects on the brain were a mystery. Recent scientific studies, however, have revealed that oxytocin plays a strong role in our ability to bond with and love one another. While all moms-to-be produce oxytocin, those who had higher levels of oxytocin during their pregnancy and postpartum months reported more loving and bonding behaviors with their babies. They also reported being more preoccupied with thoughts of checking on their babies, their infant's safety, and their baby's future. While most of us worry about our babies even when we're staring at them through our video baby monitors—and can be oh-too-easily coaxed into discussing our child's future college prospects—it's nice to be assured that we're hardwired for this behavior. Studies have also indicated that certain activities such as sex, eating dark chocolate, taking a warm shower, or a massage can increase our levels of oxytocin. So, provided your doctor approves, try a few or all of the above and think of it as a little "baby bonding medicine" and just what the doctor ordered.

I begin to love this creature, and to anticipate her birth as a fresh twist to a knot, which I do not wish to untie.

—*Mary Wollstonecraft*

Dark Chocolate Love Bark

1 (4 ounce) dark chocolate bar, broken into chunks
½ C whole toasted almonds
¼ C dried cranberries
¼ C candied ginger sliced into bite-size nibbles

Melt chocolate in a double-boiler over low heat until melted.

Add the almonds, cranberries, and ginger to the chocolate and stir. Pour chocolate mixture onto a cookie sheet lined with parchment paper.
Let bark cool completely. Break into pieces and serve.

Serves one hungry Mommy.

My Mama always said,
life is like a box of chocolates—you
never know what
you're gonna get.

—*Forrest Gump in* Forrest Gump *(1994)*

A "WHILE WE WERE WAITING FOR YOU" SCRAPBOOK

Who says birth is a prerequisite for a biography? Buck convention and record this exciting new chapter in your life with an original "bump biography" in the form of a scrapbook. It's guaranteed to become an instant classic on your family bookshelf.

JOURNAL THE JOURNEY. We know you think you'll never forget every minute detail of that big day when you found out you were expecting—the date, where you were, your first reaction, whom you told first and how—but trust us, time and sleep deprivation have a funny way of glossing over the details. So capture the momentous occasion by writing it all down. You'll be glad you did when your bump is a distant memory that's been replaced with a little person who just loves to hear how it all began.

BABY, YOU GOT AROUND. Keep little notes, ticket stubs, postcards, snapshots, and mementos of the trips, visits, and things you did while pregnant. Tuck in a menu from your favorite restaurant or even a candy wrapper from a must-have craving. Include cards and printed e-mails from family and friends or make little notes of conversations and reactions.

BABY'S READY FOR A CLOSE-UP. This is a great place to feature your ultrasound photos along with any fun notes or comments. "The doctor said you had big feet," or "Look! You were waving at us." Observations will be sweet ways to recall those anticipatory days when your little bump was so close yet seemed so far away. Be sure to include pictures of yourself and your belly at various stages. You'll be surprised at what you'll notice when you look back—that tie-dyed maternity top that seems so boho chic now will have you all in stitches years from now.

CRIB NOTES. Keep a few pages blank in your scrapbook and take it with you to your baby showers or family gatherings so people can share good wishes and advice or even doodles. This is also a great place to save your baby shower invitations and photos.

SAVE THE BEST FOR LAST. Reserve the last page for the first photo of your sweet baby on his or her birth day when a whole new chapter—a whole new baby book—will begin.

Gingerbread Patty Cakes

1 C sugar
1 C unsalted butter, melted
1 C molasses
1 C boiling water
2 tsp baking soda
Pinch of salt
2½ T powdered ginger
½ tsp cinnamon
2½ C all-purpose flour
2 eggs, beaten
¼ C powdered sugar

Preheat oven to 350 degrees. Spray muffin tin with nonstick cooking spray.

In one bowl mix together the sugar, butter, molasses, and boiling water. Set aside.

In another bowl mix together the baking soda, salt, ginger, cinnamon, and flour.

Whisk the wet ingredients into the dry ingredients. Mix in eggs. The batter will be very thin.

Pour the batter into muffin tins, filling each ¾ full.

Bake for 45 minutes or until a toothpick inserted into center of muffins comes out clean. Dust tops with powdered sugar. Makes 12 muffins.

I Know It by Heart

Much has been written about the popular "Mozart effect"—the theory that listening to classical music in utero can make your baby smarter. For those of us who already enjoy music, the news that we *should* play music for our bumps was a little like telling us chocolate milkshakes are good for us. But recent trends in rocking the womb show that mothers are playing music for their bumps not because they're trying to give them a prenatal head start, but because they know that babies recognize and remember sounds and voices from the womb.

Years ago conductor and inspirational speaker Boris Brott claimed that he recognized symphonies that his mother, a professional cellist, played while pregnant with him. While most moms can't claim to be professional cellists, many are now choosing a theme song to sway to regularly on their MP3 players with the hope that familiar music can be a source of comfort, and a way of connecting, to their baby after he's born.

Although scientists don't know exactly how much of a song or symphony your baby might be able to hear in the womb, many mothers claim that when their newborns hear "their song" they get still and appear to listen deeply.

In terms of choosing a tune—we'll leave the prenatal deejay choices to you and your bump.

Play It Again, Mom

When I was pregnant with my first son I played the piano every day, sometimes for hours. I played out my anxieties and fears as well as my joys and excitement. Our daily recitals were only interrupted when my son, Blaise, was born via C-section. The day we came home from the hospital, my mother was holding him on her chest, walking slowly around the room as he dozed. And while I was still in quite a bit of pain, I hobbled over to the bench and began to softly play a favorite song. My newborn, only days old, lifted his head from his grandmother's chest, and wide-eyed and searching, turned his head toward the music in what can only be called recognition. We were stunned at the display of strength and focus. I now have four children, and they all take piano lessons—some more enthusiastically than others—but Blaise is the only one who can play by ear. Where everyone else reads music and counts keys, Blaise has the uncanny ability to master a song with just a little exploration. The music simply pours from within him, as steady and familiar as his own heartbeat. —Marlene

Got the Music in Me

When I was pregnant with my son Hank, I was obsessed with music, or shall I say "we" were obsessed. Ordinarily, I enjoyed music, but something about being pregnant—or perhaps something about who I was pregnant with—made me literally crave it. My pregnancy was a veritable soundtrack of tunes from lullabies, top 40, and classical music to pop, gospel, and show tunes. It was a radio-blaring, CD-blasting nine-month-long concert. I literally "had the music in me." Hank came out screaming but I think it was an Aerosmith tribute. "Mama, I want a guitar I can plug into the wall," he said the other day as he strutted across the room wearing dark sunglasses, with his plastic guitar. It is never quiet around our house, and I march to the beat of violin and piano lessons and the occasional drum solo beaten out on my pots and pans. And it's all music to my ears. —Justina

⊙⊙ Postcard *to the* Bump ⊙⊙

My favorite song while you were my bump was ....
....
....
....
....

My mom is a never-ending **song in my heart** of comfort, happiness, and being. I may sometimes forget the words but **I always remember the tune.** —*Graycie Harmon*

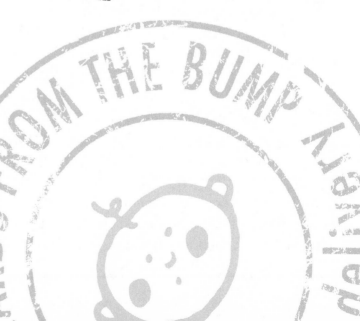

A Mother Hen Told Us...
Nothing says love like a mixtape. Create a playlist of songs for your baby that reflect the musical tastes of her parents. Rocking the cradle is so much easier when you have your very own soundtrack.

CREATING A NESTY LITTLE NOOK

Your baby is currently set up in "a womb of her own," but it's up to you to create a spot that's big and comfortable enough for the two of you to relax and rest. Think of it as a retreat for mind, body, and bump, or your very own prenatal perch—a suite spot that will be your ticket to emotional and physical comfort and a great place for Mom to take a timeout.

ME, MYSELF, AND BUMP. Stake out a quiet spot in the house, like the baby's nursery, or a quiet corner near a window, and transform it into a love nest for you and your egg. Make it as private and separate from the rest of your home as you can.

FEATHERING YOUR NESTY NOOK. Find a comfortable glider or an upholstered rocking chair. Used chairs can be found at yard sales, stores that sell used nursery items, and online. This comfy piece of furniture will be indispensable in your nursery, so invest the time and effort into finding the right one. It will get you through years of feedings, rock-a-byes, readings, and snuggles. A small, sturdy table or bookshelf pulled close will provide a place for setting a beverage as well as give handy access for stacking books and magazines.

CREATURE COMFORTS. Indulge in some items that make your space feel like a pampering retreat—an etched carafe for ice water, a pretty new teacup, a plush throw, fresh flowers, a leather-bound journal, or a juicy new novel. Accessorize sentimentally with framed family photos or a handmade quilt. Ban items that remind you of work, chores, and to-dos.

SET THE MOOD. Mama can't rock without music, so furnish your sweet spot with a speaker dock for your MP3 player, a boom box, or radio. Complete the soothing atmosphere with a delicately scented soy candle and bliss out with your bump.

MAKE IT A REGULAR RENDEZVOUS. Whether you use it to take a catnap or indulge in some easy listening, be sure to carve out some regular time to visit your nook.

ᴗᴗ Postcard *to the* Bump ᴗᴗ

I had a feeling you were going to be a boy/girl when ....

....

....

....

....

Everything grows **rounder and wider and weirder,** and I sit here in the middle of it all and wonder who in the world you will turn out to be. *—Carrie Fisher*

Boy or Girl? Old Wives' Tales and Gender Forecasting

Until the ultrasound put them out of business, old wives had a thriving gender prediction business. Take a timeout to enjoy a little old-fashioned fun with your bump and these very unscientific forecasting methods borrowed from the old wives themselves.

• If you crave salty foods, it's a boy. Sweets? It's a girl.

• If you're carrying "basketball style"—all out front, or down low—it's a boy. If you're carrying "inner tube style"—all around or up high—it's a girl.

• Present your hands to someone. If your palms are up, it's a girl. Palms down? It's a boy.

• Take the "breast test." If your left one is larger than your right, it's a girl. If the right one's bigger, it's a boy.

• Tie your wedding ring to a piece of thread and have someone hold it pendulum style over your belly. If it swings in a circle or oval, it's a girl. If it swings straight back and forth, it's a boy.

• Girls give you morning sickness; boys don't.

• If this baby's older sibling said "Da-da" first, it's a boy. If he or she said, "Ma-ma" first, it's a girl.

• If your hands are dry and rough, it's a boy. Girls give you soft and supple hands.

• Have someone roll a penny down your back. If it lands on heads, it's a boy; tails, it's a girl.

• Pick up a key. If you grabbed it by the long end, it's a girl; by the round end, it's a boy.

• If your rear view looks normal, it's a boy; if your bump is obvious even from behind you, it's a girl.

• If you like bread slices from the center of the loaf, it's a girl; if you like the heels of the bread loaf, it's a boy.

• Take your age of conception and the year you conceived. If both are even, or both are odd, it's a girl. If it's one odd and one even, it's a boy.

• Poll five five-year-olds as to whether you are having a boy or a girl. Whatever the majority says will be what you are having.

• If you like to lay on your left side, it's a boy. Right side more comfortable? It's a girl.

• Moodier than usual? It's a girl because your womanly moods are "doubled." If you are the same or more easygoing in temperament, it's a boy.

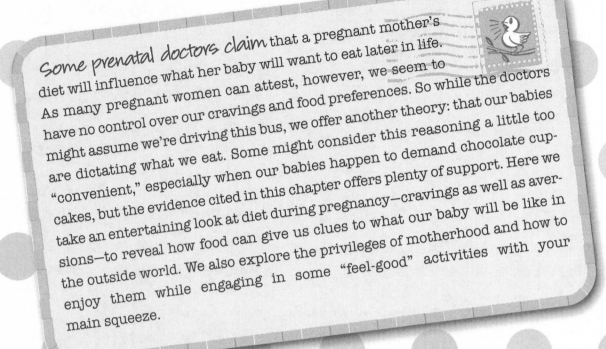

Some prenatal doctors claim that a pregnant mother's diet will influence what her baby will want to eat later in life. As many pregnant women can attest, however, we seem to have no control over our cravings and food preferences. So while the doctors might assume we're driving this bus, we offer another theory: that our babies are dictating what we eat. Some might consider this reasoning a little too "convenient," especially when our babies happen to demand chocolate cupcakes, but the evidence cited in this chapter offers plenty of support. Here we take an entertaining look at diet during pregnancy—cravings as well as aversions—to reveal how food can give us clues to what our baby will be like in the outside world. We also explore the privileges of motherhood and how to enjoy them while engaging in some "feel-good" activities with your main squeeze.

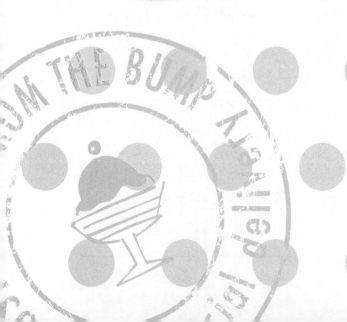

POSTCARDS FROM THE BUMP

UNLESS YOUR NAME IS BEN OR JERRY,
THERE'S ABSOLUTELY NO WAY
WE CAN FIT YOU INTO OUR
BUSY SCHEDULE TODAY.
—*Ame and Emily*

2   2

❧ CHAPTER TWO ❧

Blame it on the Bump
Who's _Really_ Craving those French Fries and Foot Rubs?

DEAR MOM, things are going swimmingly well in here. It's a little like Vegas—hard to tell day from night but I'm so cozy I don't really care. Can you believe I just perfected my triple flip? Did'ya feel it? I can't believe I got three full rotations in this tight space—just wait 'til I get on the outside. I'm ___ quadruple roll. It's gonna be sweet! LOVE YOU, the Bum___ ___ I know you can't feel me or hear me yet but I am so ___ to say "hello," soon. Forever Your Girl or Boy, the BUM___ ___ I ___ it must have bee___ ___ the person who la___ ___ ma? Oh, and I lo___ ___—I think I hear___ ___ore of that. You___ ___ ming voice and that las___ ___. And whatever you played in ___ out- standing. But that clas___ ___ ing of which, I'm way overdue for my nap so I'll catch 'ya later alligator. LOVE You! DEAR MOM, That salami sandwich with the deli dill on the side and a mango sorbet chaser was divine. Now if you would only have some cotton candy, Manchego cheese and a chocolate-chip cookie—it would be pure bliss! I'm getting a little tired of vanilla ice cream, though—how 'bout busting out with a little Rocky Road? LOVE U, the Bump ...DEAR

A Burning Love

Long before I could ever legitimately claim I was "eating for two," I was a serial eater prone to food infatuations that consumed me for months at a time. And, I confess to a lengthy love affair with nachos that ended very badly.

I was smitten with the kind of nachos that you can find only at high school concession stands or county fairs, where they scoop chips from five-pound bags and glowing yellow sauce from barrels. When I asked my husband if we could invest in the commercial ingredients to keep at home, he replied, "Honey, there's

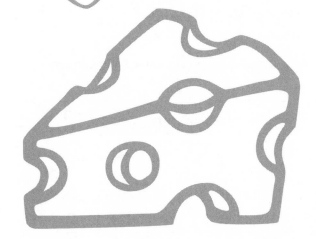

no way you can eat 128 ounces of cheese sauce before it goes bad."

"But I've got four years before it expires," I'd retort.

After weeks of careful experimentation, I finally came up with a healthier variation that didn't require a restaurant license, a pickup truck, or a home addition to manage the ingredients. I ignored my husband's complaints that our house smelled like a bowling alley and his comments that "anything that dries that hard in a bowl can't be good for you."

One night after an hour at the gym (a sacrifice I willingly made to counter the effects of my high-calorie liaison), I rushed home to get things cooking. I was so hot for my tryst that I used the microwave instead of the usual stovetop preparation. With oven mitts I pulled the bubbling concoction from the microwave and carried the sauce into the living room, a bag of tortilla chips dangling from my teeth. Steps away from the couch, the plastic bowl, weakened by the scorching heat, imploded. Molten hot cheese sauce ran down my body, scalding my feet and pooling into the carpet, where it quickly began to congeal. It took countless hand-chapping scrub sessions to clean up the disgusting muck while my husband stood over me like a wicked, disapproving stepmother, hands on hips, shaking his head. The sour smell lingered for months—a nasty reminder of the traumatic end of my cheesy affair.

Then one beautiful autumn day, six months pregnant, I was waddling around a harvest festival when a smell from the past exploded in my nose, triggering fireworks of pleasure in my brain. The scent ignited such longing that my feet seemed to lift from the ground, and like a balloon on a string, the aroma tugged me along until I found myself standing in front of a nacho cart.

It was a blissful reunion that included my new little love, who seemed to enjoy nachos as much as I did. She'd kick and roll in my belly as I precariously balanced a plate of tortilla chips, smothered in cheese and jalapenos, on my bump.

Eventually, our social outings began to revolve around my renewed nacho addiction. "Wanna go to a baseball game?" my husband would ask.

"You mean go eat nachos? Sure," I'd reply.

My husband teased that we should name the baby Chip.

"Not a good idea," I countered. "I might eat her."

After our daughter was born, my fiery passion for nachos abruptly cooled to something more platonic. Much as one feels about a nice ex-boyfriend, I didn't hate them, but I could happily wave and walk right by without a twinge of pining. They say old lovers can never be good friends, but when my seven-year-old daughter begs for nachos and I spoon that gooey concoction over chips, I can't help but feel a deep affection for my old flame.

The belly rules the mind.

—Spanish proverb

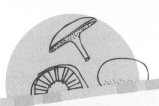

Sweet Potato Before I became pregnant, I always thought that the "cravings" women claimed to have were just an excuse to eat whatever crazy stuff they wanted without judgment. So no one was more amazed than I when, during my third month, I began to gravitate to a new favorite food—potatoes. A few months later the craving was so strong that a friend brought over a potato-themed gift basket in my honor. My bump, Kendall, seemed to be emulating our new craving and spent most days lazing and floating around, which made the "kick counts" of late pregnancy a little nerve-racking. After she was born, she remained an easygoing baby and was a very late walker. Today, at nine years old, you will most likely find her curled up on the couch with a book, and her favorite food is, of course, baked potatoes! —Caroline

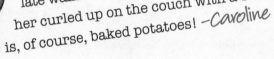

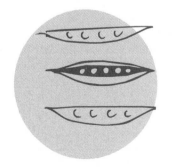

✍ Postcard *to the* Bump ✍

Our favorite food was ....

....

....

....

HOT, SWEET, OR TANGY?
What Flavor Is Your Bump?

Which came first—the chick jonesing for ice cream or a little egg with a demanding sweet tooth? The latter may not be so far-fetched, after all. Studies have shown that your bump can actually "taste" what you're eating since your food choices "flavor" your amniotic fluid. So who's to say those cravings aren't your bump's creative way of ordering up more of his or her own favorites?

At about week 12, babies begin to swallow the amniotic fluid that surrounds them, so it figures that their taste buds would develop soon thereafter—around 13–15 weeks. In watching ultrasounds, researchers noted that babies opened their mouths and stuck out their tongues as if they were "tasting" the amniotic fluid. Sure enough, they later documented that babies swallowed more fluid when the mothers had eaten sweet foods and ingested less, and actually made faces in response to the fluid when Mom had dined on something bitter or sour.

By the last trimester, babies swallow over four cups of amniotic fluid a day, which leads some to speculate that the flavored fluid is serving as an "appetizer" for the main course to come: breast milk—which also happens to be flavored by a mother's dietary choices. These in utero food preferences have also been shown to carry over after birth. For instance, babies who had "tasted" carrots in utero, thanks to Mom's regularly drinking carrot juice, liked carrots much more than babies whose mothers didn't drink the orange stuff.

Tell me what you eat,
I'll tell you who you are.

—*Anthelme Brillat-Savarin*

BABY BUILDING BLOCKS: EATING WELL WHILE YOU'RE SWELL

Pregnant or not, most of us attempt to eat a healthy, balanced diet, but when you're eating for two, you have yet another giant reason to pay attention to what goes in your mouth and, eventually, into your baby. Generally, the average woman needs to up her calorie intake by about only 300 calories a day when pregnant. Calorie requirements hinge on whether you are underweight, overweight, just right, or carrying more than one baby—so run your specific needs by your doctor. High-quality calories from nutrient-rich foods are the best "baby foods," but eating well as your belly swells need not be difficult. Here are some simple foods that are good for you both.

EGGS: Rich in protein, choline, and omega-3, eggs are essentially baby brain food.

CHICKEN: A lean source of protein, chicken is the perfect way to fortify your little egg.

MILK: Build yours and your baby's bones with calcium. Nonfat milk skimps on calories but not calcium, but the richness of whole milk can help you put on weight if you need to gain.

LEGUMES: Rich in fiber and protein and lean in fat, beans really count when you are pregnant. Black-eyed peas, chick peas, navy beans, split peas, kidney beans, black beans—they all add up to healthy eating.

STRING CHEESE: This calcium-rich toddler favorite is good for your bump before he even gets here.

RAISINS: These little treats are perfect for on-the-go snacking and pack a lot of nutrition in a little package. Raisins give you iron, fiber, and even a little bit of protein.

YOGURT: Calcium-rich and chock full of healthy enzymes that can boost digestive health, yogurt is an easy snack for grab-and-go nutrition. Up the benefits with a sprinkling of almonds, raisins, or fresh berries.

LEAFY GREENS: Filled with iron, fiber, and beta

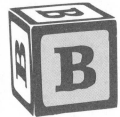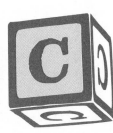

carotene, leafy green veggies like cabbage, spinach, lettuce, and collard greens are great for you both.

WHOLE GRAIN BREADS: Chock full of fiber, complex carbohydrates for energy, and a good source of the B vitamin and folic acid, bread is good for bumps.

BABY CARROTS: Surprisingly sweet and satisfying, baby carrots are an easy way to pack in some beta carotene, fiber, and vitamin A. Pair them with Preggy Veggie Dip (see recipe on p. 142) for a delicious snack.

FORTIFIED BRAN CEREAL—Just 3/4 of a cup of most fortified cereals contains 100 percent of your daily folate needs. In addition to folic acid, bran-rich cereals will help keep things moving comfortably along the digestive tract.

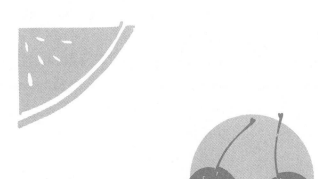

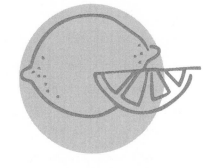

Mama Hen Cabbage Salad

For the dressing:
¼ C rice wine vinegar
¼ tsp red pepper flakes
¼ C cabbage mix
2 T toasted sesame seeds
2 T peanut butter
1 clove of garlic, sliced thin

1 rotisserie chicken, shredded
1 tsp sesame oil
1 bag slaw mix (about 4 cups; reserve ¼ C for dressing)
½ C chopped peanuts for garnish

For the dressing: Puree all ingredients in a blender until smooth; set aside.

In a large bowl, toss the shredded chicken with sesame oil, then toss in the cabbage mix and dressing.

Serve on a platter. Garnish with chopped peanuts.

Raisin' Baby Bran Muffins

2 C Raisin Bran cereal
½ tsp salt
2½ C whole wheat flour
½ tsp baking soda
2 T flax seed
1 C sugar
¼ C canola oil
¼ C apple sauce
2 eggs, beaten
½ quart buttermilk
1 C dried cranberries

Preheat oven to 400 degrees.

Combine dry ingredients, then stir in oil, apple sauce, eggs, buttermilk, and cranberries. Let batter rest for half an hour. Pour into muffin tin or muffin cups.

Bake at 400 degrees for 20 minutes. Makes 24 mini muffins or 12 regular-size muffins.

Sweet Mama-Mia Tortillas

1 large whole wheat tortilla
2 T peanut butter
¼ C shelled sunflower seeds
¼ C raisins
1 banana, peeled

Flatten out the tortilla and spread with peanut butter. Sprinkle with sunflower seeds and raisins. Place banana at one end and roll the tortilla up around the banana. Cut into bite-size pieces.

Bump Bonus

Feeling the baby move for the first time."

"Telling my mom she was *finally* going to be a grandmother."

"Falling asleep with my husband's hand on my belly."

My friends fired back their answers to the question: "What was your favorite part about being pregnant?" at dinner one night. As the wave of emotion swept around the table, I noticed one friend, Carrie, squirming in her chair, looking anything but eager for the query to roll around to her. The more sweet recollections the group offered up, the more uncomfortable she looked. When it was her turn, she met our eager faces with a sheepish grin.

"Okay, okay. Don't judge me," she said and, with her hand covering her mouth, mumbled, "Cole Haan high heels."

"What?" several of us asked.

"Shoes," she blurted out. "My favorite thing about being pregnant was this awesome pair of shoes I splurged on. The baby needed them—they made us feel so good!"

For a brief moment there was silence.

"Ben and Jerry's Chubby Hubby with caramel sauce every night," Linda blurted out, filling the pause. "That's what I *really* wanted to say."

"Lying on the couch while Bob washed the dishes and folded laundry," another confessed.

"Obsessing over the perfect shade of pink for the nursery," someone added.

"The boobs—that bra-busting cleavage was amazing."

The profound moments, the *big* things, of pregnancy are truly sublime, but Carrie's honesty had unleashed a verbal surge on the more superficial perks and indulgences of our pregnancies and all the little things we relished. Like the foods—sandwiches with sweet pickles and cream cheese, salami and anchovies on crackers, black jelly beans with peanuts. And the hedonistic: foot rubs on demand, a weekend at the spa, chocolate-covered strawberries.

We had started this rare evening of "Mommy's night out" with a "no baby talk" vow, but how quickly the fertile common ground of pregnancy had sucked us in. The shared drama of having children proved too irresistible a topic for a circle of women with babies at home. Like the chardonnay we were indulging in, reminiscing over our bumps left a mellow, deeply satisfying taste in our mouths, but our confessions made those memories bubble and pop like champagne!

Postcard *to the* Bump

Some of my favorite things about being pregnant were

....

....

....

....

....

....

Kicking Back I was working as a teacher when I was pregnant with my son Matt and one day at recess, a kick ball came flying out of nowhere and smacked me squarely in the belly. It took a trip to the hospital and an ultrasound to calm me down. Thankfully a pregnant belly provides wonderful cushiony, protection and we were both fine. Unlike me, my bump seemed quite excited by his close encounter with the ball and so began a kicking-fest that lasted throughout the rest of my pregnancy. Sometimes I'd worry that he was kicking in defense or trauma but then it would feel like he was simply having fun. We got our answer when our little "Beckham" walked onto the soccer field for the first time. All those months had simply been practice as he seems to have been born a soccer star! —*Jennifer*

Love and pregnancy
and riding on a camel
cannot be hid. —*Arab Proverb*

❧ Postcard *to the* Bump ❧

My favorite maternity outfit consisted of ....
....
....
....
....
....

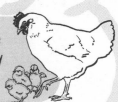

A Mother Hen Told Us... Since your body retains more fluid during pregnancy, the cliché of craving pickles could be nature's way of getting you to eat more salt to help balance out sodium levels.

Super Sniffer I love lavender and have it in every form imaginable—dryer sachets, drawer liners, soaps, wreaths, laundry detergent, candles, home fragrance diffusers, body mist, bath oil—if it can be scented with lavender essential oil, I've got it. When I became pregnant, friends warned me that my beloved lavender might not smell so sweet. Averse to lavender? I couldn't bear the thought. As predicted, pregnancy did bump up my sense of smell to bionic proportions, but it only supercharged my love for lavender. What had once been a lovely aromatherapy experience became euphoric. I even took lavender soy candles to burn in my hospital room when I delivered my son. Now as a toddler he shares my lavender infatuation and insists on deeply sniffing everything from food to flowers. On walks he makes sure I always stop to smell the roses—what a sweet teacher I gave birth to. —*Eliza*

Postcard *to the* Bump

I loved the smell of ....
....
....
....
....
....
....
....

The flower is the
poetry of reproduction.
It is an example of the eternal
seductiveness of life. —*Jean Giraudoux*

LOVE'S BABY SOFT:
Follow Your Nose

Surprisingly, by week 28 your baby can smell almost everything you eat or inhale. From Grandma's mouthwatering lasagna to Daddy's aftershave, your bump is savoring the smells of the outside world. Just like taste, smells are transferred to your baby through your amniotic fluid. According to scientists, some scents are even enhanced by your amniotic fluid, and your baby's activities, such as swallowing, help to circulate the odors through your womb. These smells allow your baby to familiarize herself with the odors of the outside world from food aromas to basic household scents. Yet even more important than the scent of chocolate cookies is "eau de Mommy" because your amniotic fluid smells a lot like you, too—which means that your amazing kiddo can sniff you out of a crowd. If that's somewhat intimidating, don't fret, because recent studies have shown that we moms also share that skill; mothers who have spent as little as ten minutes with their newborns are able to correctly identify their young one's clothing by smell alone.

Angels must surely smell of baby powder.

—*Anonymous*

Bump Berries Grapes. My mouth waters just thinking about them. With my first two pregnancies I bought two pounds of grapes practically every day. I'd wash them, display them prettily in a bowl on my desk under the guise of "sharing" them with my coworkers, then proceed to eat every single one myself. Even in the throes of morning sickness, grapes still tasted good to me. Both those grape-loving bumps have grown into kids who still adore grapes by the pound. —Kristin

The 12-step chocoholics program: Never be more than 12 steps away from chocolate.

—*Terry Moore*

My mother was actually eating French fries when she went into labor with me. I'm a grown woman with two children of my own, but French fries remain my **all-time favorite food**.

—*Jennifer Mitchell*

Taking Candy from a Mama My first two bumps craved fruit—healthy, juicy, Mother Nature sweets that I guiltlessly put away by the pounds. I felt like a healthy "green goddess" and would tsk-tsk at my friends who were in bondage to pints of pecan praline ice cream and bags of M&Ms. When they'd bemoan their weight gain, I'd suggest they trade in the candy for fruit, and I never understood the blank stares I got . . . until I became pregnant with baby number three. Aiden, as my bump was later named, turned me into a raving chocoholic. Chocolate cake, chocolate-chip cookies, chocolate ice cream, and yes, M&Ms—ruled my days. To this day I'm devastated if I don't get my daily chocolate fix—and Aiden is right there with me. –Kristin

Does a box of
Milk Duds
count as a serving
of calcium?
—*Beth Teitell*

I'd stuff myself with **cookies all morning**—whatever was in the cupboard, really—then I'd have a box of **Krispy Kreme doughnuts** for dessert. And I once ate two whole packs of coffee cake in one sitting!
—*Milla Jovovich*

Goo-Goo Ga-Ga Cookies

½ C (1 stick) butter, softened
⅓ C peanut butter, smooth
⅓ C sugar
⅓ C light brown sugar, packed
1 egg
1 tsp vanilla
1¼ C all-purpose flour
½ tsp baking soda
1 package (12 ounces) semisweet chocolate chips
1 C chopped pecans
24 pecan halves

Preheat oven to 350 degrees. Line two cookie sheets with parchment paper or Silpat liners.

Beat butter, peanut butter, sugars, egg, and vanilla in large bowl until fluffy.
Combine flour and baking soda and add into wet ingredients.

Stir in chocolate chips and pecans.
Use a small, spring-loaded ice-cream scoop to place balls of dough on cookie sheets, spacing about three inches apart. Press a pecan half on top of each cookie to flatten slightly.

Bake 15 to 17 minutes or until firm in center. Remove to wire racks to cool. Makes about 3 dozen cookies.

Chocolate "Bun in the Oven" Bread Pudding

1 T butter, plus more for baking dish
10 slices cinnamon-raisin bread, crusts removed
2 C milk
¼ C semisweet chocolate chips
2 large eggs
½ C sugar
½ tsp vanilla extract
Confectioner's sugar for dusting

Preheat oven to 350 degrees. Coat a nine-inch square baking dish with cooking spray; set aside. Lightly toast the bread.

Combine milk, chocolate, and butter in a saucepan over medium-low heat. Stir occasionally, until chocolate melts.

Tear each slice of bread into four or five pieces and stack evenly on the bottom of the buttered baking dish. Whisk together the eggs, granulated sugar, and vanilla in a medium bowl. Add the warm milk mixture and whisk until combined. Pour mixture evenly over the bread.

Bake for 25 minutes until pudding is firm and puffed up. Let it cool for 15 minutes, then dust each serving with confectioner's sugar.

Souper Recipes

Sometimes all a pregnant tummy can handle is a bowl of satisfying soup. Serve with some hot fresh bread and enjoy!

Broccoli Cheese Soup

3 medium bunches of broccoli, chopped
½ C butter
1 medium onion, chopped
2 garlic cloves, crushed
½ C flour
2 C milk
48-ounce can of low-sodium chicken broth
Salt and pepper to taste
1½ C cheddar cheese, grated

Steam broccoli until tender. Transfer broccoli to food processor and puree lightly.

Sauté onions in butter for five minutes. Stir in milk, flour, garlic, salt, and pepper. Stir in grated cheese and blend until smooth. Slowly stir in chicken broth. Add broccoli puree slowly, stirring until well blended. Simmer for 15 minutes, or longer for thicker soup.
Serves 6 to 8.

Potato Leek Soup

Two leeks, diced (white and light green parts)
3–4 medium potatoes, diced
Medium onion, chopped
4 T butter
4 C vegetable stock
2½ C milk
Pepper and salt to taste

Cook first three ingredients in four tablespoons of butter in a saucepan over medium heat for about ten minutes or until they start to soften. Then slowly add four cups of vegetable stock. Slowly add 1/2 cup of milk. Let mixture simmer about 30 minutes, then in batches put it in the blender and purée until smooth. Return soup to the stove and slowly stir in the remaining two cups milk and pepper and salt to taste. Let simmer until ready to eat.
Serves 4 to 6.

Spicy Pumpkin Soup

1/2 C butter
2 large onions, chopped
4 garlic cloves, crushed
1 T curry powder
1 tsp salt
½ tsp coriander
½ tsp crushed red pepper
2 quarts chicken broth
3 C half and half
5½ C solid packed pumpkin (canned)

Melt butter in saucepan. Sauté onions and garlic until soft. Add curry, salt, coriander, and red pepper and cook for five minutes over medium heat. Add broth slowly and simmer 15 minutes. Gradually stir in half and half. Heat through and add pumpkin. Stir well until blended. Transfer soup into blender in batches. Blend until creamy. Return soup to the stove; let it simmer until you're ready to eat. Serves: 6 to 8.

A Mother Hen Told Us... When you cook a soup, double the recipe and freeze half for later. Before placing it in the refrigerator or freezer, let your soup cool completely and store it in a moisture-proof, freezer-safe container. Leave about a quarter inch of room in the container for expansion and label and date your soup. Eat within two months of freezing.

OOOO BABY, BABY

Feel-good, sensual, soul-stirring touch: We all know how good touch makes us feel and—news flash—you didn't get that bump from keeping your hands to yourself. We're born with the need for physical contact; in fact, touch is the first of our senses to develop, just shy of the eighth week of gestation. From that first tingle, a baby is cradled in the constant sensation of warmth against her skin and the buoyant feeling of being rocked by a mother's movements. It's no wonder that newborns love to be held, caressed, and swaddled—and let's face it, so do

we. Healing touch has many physical and emotional benefits aside from the obvious—it can reduce stress and anxiety, relieve muscle pain, increase blood flow to reduce swelling, and help you get a better night's sleep. Check with your doctor and find a prescription for babying yourself that includes a big dose of healing, restorative touch, such as those listed below:

PREGNANCY MASSAGE. It may not be your first trip to the spa, but now that you have a bump it's

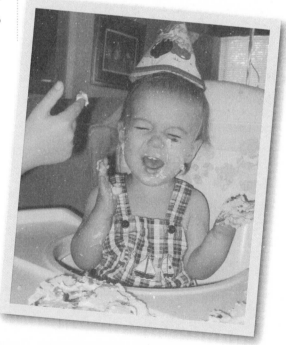

At a tender age,
Luke discovered that
STRESSED is indeed
DESSERTS
spelled backwards.

a whole new ballgame. Just because you're pregnant and you want a massage does not make for a pregnancy massage. Be sure to put yourself and your baby in good hands—a certified pregnancy massage therapist who has been specially trained on the anatomy and specific needs of pregnant women. As tempting as those massage tables with a hole in the middle may seem, avoid them. We know it seems like a good idea, but suspending your belly through a hole can be uncomfortable or even dangerous since the position can cause undo stress on your lower back, joints, and muscles. Pregnancy is the perfect time to indulge in massage—you've got double the reasons to find someone to rub you the right way.

REFLEXOLOGY. Grounded in an ancient form of healing, reflexology is based on the belief that specific areas in your feet, hands, and ears called "reflex zones" mirror certain organs, glands, and other areas of the body and that massaging or stretching these reflex zones promotes healing in the corresponding spots. Fans of reflexology tout benefits from increased energy and morning-sickness relief to reduction of swelling and heartburn. Consult with your doctor first to find a reflexologist with pregnancy certification. We think anything that involves a foot rub is worth a shot.

ACUPRESSURE. Often described as acupuncture without the needles, acupressure is a centuries-old Chinese healing art that believes in balancing the life force, or "chi," by manipulating meridian points on the body through touch. In place of needles, acupressurists apply pressure to these points on the body's surface using their fingers, elbows, and hands. Some women swear by its restorative properties for everything from relaxation and mood elevation to inducing labor and pain relief. Again, get your doctor's okay and see an acupressurist who has pregnancy training. All of a sudden being under pressure doesn't sound like such a bad idea!

A BUMPY START:
For Those about to Hurl

Don't you just love people who tell you that a little of this or a little of that can stop your morning sickness forever? It's ever so helpful to listen to their lectures when all you really need to do is run to the john and toss your cookies. We're not going to mince words here. There is no cure for morning sickness—which really should be renamed round-the-clock barf-o-rama. If you suffer, you're not alone since it affects about 70 percent of pregnant women and usually begins around week 4 and ends around week 16. Though scientists aren't sure of the exact cause of morning sickness (thankfully, pregnant women don't make great lab rats), they speculate that it's brought on by the surge of hormones that help protect your growing fetus.

Here are some tips from both researchers and smart mamas that, while not guaranteed to cure

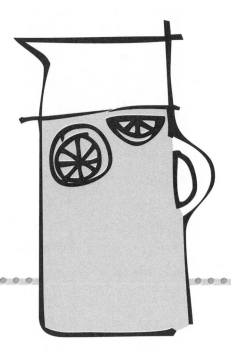

A Mother Hen Told Us...
Keep a tin of your favorite mints in your bag and give them a sniff whenever an offending smell triggers morning-sickness nausea. According to old wives' tales, the smell of peppermint is a classic remedy for calming an upset stomach.

you completely, might make it so that you don't feel like upchucking every hour of the day:

ADOPT A TASTING-MENU APPROACH TO FOOD. Serve yourself smaller portions more often throughout the day to avoid getting too hungry or too full, which can jump-start nausea. Cart around some of your favorite snacks (see p. 67) and crackers so that you never get stuck on empty.

AND IN THE FIRST TRIMESTER SHE RESTED. Reduce your list of scheduled activities, slow down and give yourself more time to sleep, and put your feet up. Researchers have found that nausea is exacerbated by not getting enough rest.

AVOID CERTAIN FOODS OR SMELLS. From the fish market to Aunt Esmer- alda's mushroom casserole, use your pregnant status as a get-outta-here-free card whenever the aromas get a little too much for you.

WANT SOME CANDY? Stock up on your favorite hard candy—lemon and ginger are preferred flavors of pregnant connoisseurs.

DRINK ME. Hydrate yourself with liquids all day long. If you know you'll be running around all day, be sure to pack yourself a water bottle.

CHECK WITH YOUR DOCTOR. These days your doctor can prescribe a safe antinausea pill that, in severe cases, may be the only thing that will help. As plenty of moms we talked to will attest, it can make all the difference if you're in a world of hurt.

. . . AND THIS LITTLE PREGGY
Ate Roast Beef

From black olives, Kentucky Fried Chicken®, and eggplant pizza to graham crackers, chocolate, and green apples, the cravings of pregnant women are as plentiful and diverse as the people on our planet. Regardless of culture, race, economics, and class, food cravings and aversions are a phenomenon shared by a staggering majority of pregnant women. In a recent study, 85 percent of expectant women polled expressed sudden, overpowering cravings or aversions to certain foods. So why the sudden hankerings once you're knocked up? Science has yet to explain the mystery, but there are many theories.

CALORIES. Put simply, you need to eat more when your body is working 'round the clock to grow another human being, so those cravings may simply be nature's way of getting you to eat more.

NUTRITION. Part old wives' tale and part medical speculation, some cravings are blamed on the specific nutritional needs brought on by pregnancy. A sudden craving for steak could signal a need for iron or protein, or an insatiable urge for oranges could help you pack in some extra vitamin C. Your body's demand for certain nutrient-rich foods could also explain why women suddenly crave something that they would never ordinarily find appetizing. Sudden aversions to bitter or sour foods could be a primitive survival instinct left over from our hunting-and-gathering days when accidentally eating a poisonous plant or fruit was a dangerous possibility.

HORMONES. Who hasn't hankered for something salty, something sweet, or both at a certain time of the month? Just as many women report cravings around their menstrual cycle, the same could be said of pregnancy when hormone levels also are in flux.

COMFORT. Certain foods are linked to happy occasions or celebrations from our past, so eating them sparks a sentimental connection that's particularly comforting to a mother's heart and tummy. Whether it's macaroni and cheese, apple pie, meatloaf, or ice cream—it's perfectly natural to crave the feel-good foods of your own childhood when you've got a bun in the oven.

WEIGHT! I Can't Have a 35 Pound Baby?!

According to the Guinness Book of World Records the biggest baby ever born tipped the scales at about 23 pounds, so our little innocents bear very little blame for most of the pounds we pack on for pregnancy. But hey, making a person is a heavy responsibility. Here's an average of how the weight stacks up (the baby's extra).

7–8 pounds • "maternal stores" of fat, protein, and other nutrients

4 pounds • blood

4 pounds • other bodily fluids

2 pounds • increase in breast size

2 pounds • amniotic fluid

2–2.5 pounds • uterus

1–2 pounds • placenta

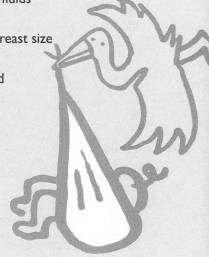

I still haven't seen my flat belly. But hell, it carried a baby! Love your own body for what it can do— say, running a 5k or dancing all night—and you won't stress as much over its wobbly bits. —*Christine Coppa*

Famous Food Cravings

You may have more in common with Angelina or Madonna than you thought. Seems that superstars are just like the rest of us when it comes to pregnancy noshing!

CHRISTINA AGUILERA—Pastries

JESSICA ALBA—Ham and cheese sandwiches

HALLE BERRY—Pepperoncinis

VICTORIA BECKHAM—Smoked salmon

CATE BLANCHETT—Pickles, ice cream

CHARLOTTE CHURCH—Pizza

DREA DE MATTEO—Italian food

MINNIE DRIVER—Olives

MAGGIE GYLLENHAAL—Tiramisu

ELISABETH HASSELBECK—Cheese, chocolate, watermelon with salt and lime

SALMA HAYEK—Chocolate

KATIE HOLMES—Cupcakes

ANGELINA JOLIE—In-N-Out® French fries dipped in milkshakes, onion rings with mustard, chocolate

NICOLE KIDMAN—Radishes

HEIDI KLUM—Ice cream

JENNIFER LOPEZ—Salsa, M&Ms®, orange soda

MADONNA—Poached eggs

DEBRA MESSING—Frosted Mini-Wheats cereal

GWYNETH PALTROW—Banana toffee pie, biscuits

SARAH JESSICA PARKER—Hamburgers, French fries

JULIA ROBERTS—Pasta

REBECCA ROMIJN—Ice cream

KERI RUSSELL—Yogurt

ASHLEE SIMPSON—Pickles and olives

TORI SPELLING—Rocky Road ice cream, avocados

GWEN STEFANI—Spicy food

CATHERINE ZETA-JONES—Marmite

❧ Postcard *to the* Bump ❧

I craved
....
....
....
....
....

MOTHERHOOD HAS ITS PRIVILEGES

No one ever says that being a mom is easy, but all that hard work and sacrifice does come with some pretty nice perks. Bump things up first class and take full advantage of your VIP (Very Important Preggy) status.

RULE THE ROOST. Now that you're an official bump-carrying member of the mother club, it's time to start trying out those four magic, maternal words: "Because I said so." If anyone dares question your attempts to pull rank, be sure to remind them that growing a person is no small feat and that given the volatility of hormones it would be ill-advised to push your buttons. Comfort is key to this club, so don't be afraid to ask firmly and sweetly for what you need.

BUMPS NEED WATER, AND LOTS OF IT. Hydration is paramount for pregnant women. Your blood volume will double by 28 weeks, amniotic fluid replenishes itself at the rate of about a cup an hour, your body's filtration systems are working overtime . . . do we really need to go on? Carry that water bottle with pride and demand unlimited refills, lemon slices, and crushed ice if you like. It's also another reason you need to pay particular attention to the next tip.

THE PRINCESS NEEDS TO PEE. Easy bathroom access is nonnegotiable at this time. Whether it's an aisle seat on an airplane, a detailed pit-stop schedule for a long car ride, or simply asking for help in scoping out the nearest bathroom at a concert or ballgame, don't be embarrassed to pay big attention to this most basic need. When you have to plead to cut in line for the ladies' room or sneak into the men's, do so graciously and shamelessly.

IS IT TIME TO EAT? Don't let the lettuce-nibbling meal-skipping set interfere with your need to eat well for two. In addition to nourishing yourself and junior, eating regular healthy meals helps stabilize your blood sugar and moods. You are building a baby, fueling his development with your nutrition—make it good! Keep your friends close and your snacks closer—carry a stash of tasty nibbles for those between-meal pinches.

TAKE A SEAT. Standing for long periods can cause leg cramps and back pain, so when that kind person offers up a bus seat don't be shy—take it. When that rude person doesn't budge from a seat, politely ask if they'd mind your sitting in their lap since you're feeling a wee bit dizzy. It's amazing how bold you can be when you remind yourself you're doing it for your baby, not just yourself.

Late to the Rodeo. When I was expecting our first child, Katelyn, my husband was a professional bronc rider, so we traveled all the time to rodeos. When I was eight months pregnant we headed out for a long truck ride to an event, but we failed to calculate my potty breaks into the travel schedule. Needless to say he barely made it to his rodeo event in time, and we'll never forgot the announcer's voice booming over the arena that Brit was late because his pregnant wife "stopped at every bathroom from Alabama to Arkansas." His embarrassment was tempered by winning the event, but from then on we left for every trip two hours early! And the little bump that had to hit every pit stop? She still loves to be on the go and we're not sure if she'll some day outgrow it, but she never lets a rest stop pass her by. —Kelli

Red Bull for Bumps

Nutritious and satisfying snacks are just what the bump ordered, and eating smaller portions more frequently will help you stay energized and avoid getting too hungry and then too full. Stock up on these ingredients so you'll be ever ready to whip out these delectable nibbles.

Sliced Apples with a dollop of peanut butter

Edamame beans sprinkled with a bit of salt (you can find them frozen in your freezer aisle)

Whole wheat pita with hummus

Roma or baby tomatoes dipped in pesto or drizzled in olive oil and balsamic vinegar

Baby carrots with bleu-cheese dressing

Sliced watermelon and grapes

Blueberries with sour cream and brown sugar

Daddy and Me Time

Your back aches, your belly's twitching, and the man half responsible for all this is watching the game with his feet up. Dads can feel—and act—a little helpless when it comes to pregnancy, but gently let him know how very much you and the bump need him. You're experiencing your baby from the inside out, and his vantage point from the outside in makes things a little harder to see. Draw him in with some touchy-feely exercises.

RUB-A-DUB-DADDY. Much to our disappointment, neither of our husbands ran out and became licensed pregnancy massage therapists when they found out we were expecting. But we didn't let their lack of experience keep them from doing some of their best amateur work. Butter him up sweetly and let him know how absolutely divine it feels when he rubs your aching feet. Explain to him that massage can stimulate blood flow and thereby reduce swelling, so it's really like he'll be "playing doc-tor." If you've got a really touching guy, look into couples massage classes for expectant parents and tell him you love it when he can't keep his hands off of you.

BABY DADDY'S GOTTA DATE. Goodbye honeymoon, hello babymoon. While your little bun is baking, it's never going to be easier to take it on the road to relish a little Mommy-Daddy bonding. Whether it's simply a weekly dinner date or an indulgent getaway (check out p. 17 for some inspiration), let him know that he'll always be your number-one man and there's no one else you'd rather be sharing this bump with.

LET HIM SUCK UP. He really may not have noticed that you can't tie your own shoes, much less scrub the bathroom floor. Give him the benefit of the doubt, but do let him know how depleting the domestic chores can be on you and how loving it feels when he vacuums the floor, folds the laundry, cooks dinner, washes the dishes, takes out the trash, dusts the furniture, pays the bills, trims the hedges, and mows the lawn. And, oh-yeah . . . no going near that nasty kitty litter for nine months!

PAT THE BELLY. "Here. She's moving. Put your hand here." The second his hand comes in contact with the surface of your skin, the little bugger stops moving. Getting him to feel the baby move can seem like an exercise in futility, but instead of putting him on the spot every ten minutes, cozy up on the couch and let him rest his hand on your belly while you watch a movie. Having a snack or a cold drink can sometimes motivate your bump to get busy. The longer the contact, the more likely he is to really get a kick out of the little one.

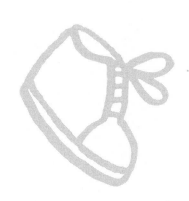

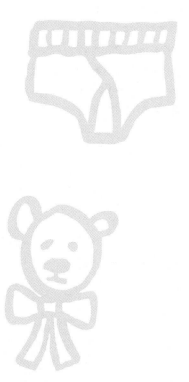

Swimming with the Endorphins

Endorphins—euphoria-inducing neurotransmitters linked to good-time pursuits like sex, chocolate, strenuous exercise (the famed "runner's high"), and massage—can now add pregnancy to the list. In 2003 a group of Michigan researchers discovered that increased estrogen levels, which soar during pregnancy, resulted in an increase in the brain's receptivity to endorphins. Being pregnant is like fishing with a bigger net when it comes to endorphins—a lot more get pulled in. We don't want to look a gift horse in the mouth, but researchers suspect the endorphin-to-estrogen equation helps moderate labor pain, since estrogen levels spike dramatically before giving birth. Just another reason to give that big belly a hug (and generate a few more endorphins while you're at it).

A great joy
is coming.
—*Anonymous*

❧ Postcard *to the* Bump ❧

Your Dad connected with you by ....
....
....
....
....
....

If you really love your wife, her pregnancy is a time to test your attention span. You have to pay attention when she says, "It's moving! Wake up and feel it!" You have to respond as if she's pointing out a replay of a touchdown pass. —*Bill Cosby*

You Want to Eat What!?

The craving for nonfood items such as dirt, soap, clay, ash, wood, starch, chalk, baking soda, and so on during pregnancy is called *pica*, the Latin word for magpie, a bird known for its indiscriminate eating habits. Old wives' tales swear that such cravings herald some sort of dietary deficiency or unmet need, but doctors are often mystified by the bizarre cravings. Some women claim that it's about the texture of the item more so than the taste; others have absolutely no explanation for their sudden urges to gnaw tree branches or lick chalkboards. One thing is for sure: You should never give into pica cravings and always tell your doctor—trust us, you're not going to shock her.

From Sweet Pea to Little Pumpkin: How Big Is Baby Now?

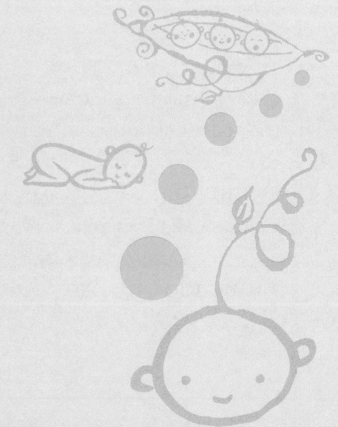

6 weeks • peppercorn

7 weeks • sweet pea

8 weeks • cherry

9 weeks • queen olive

12 weeks • kiwi

16 weeks • russet potato

20 weeks • eggplant

24 weeks • acorn squash

28 weeks • large zucchini

32 weeks • cantaloupe

36 weeks • icebox watermelon

40 weeks • pumpkin

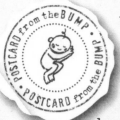

Have a Cookie When I was pregnant with my daughter, Jill, I had a very strong craving for an ordinary cookie—a sugar cookie made by a grocery-store brand, Mothers. I'd eat them every chance I got and any time—day or night. Recently Jill called me to say, "Mom, you know what I'm in the mood to eat?" Of course I guessed right—she still loves those cookies nearly 40 years later! I like to think that she was somehow telling me to eat them when she was in my belly. *—Karen*

Honestly, **only olives.** That's all I really dream about. I dream about **enormous olives.**

—Minnie Driver

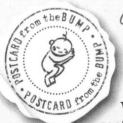

Cilantro When I was pregnant with Jacob, I had the strangest, sudden craving—cilantro. It was like catnip for a cat—I'd smell it while walking through the produce section of the grocery aisle, and I'd have to rub my face in it. I would add it to anything I could—even sandwiches. After Jacob was born I forgot all about it, as the craving was gone. Then one day when Jacob was about four, I made a soup with cilantro in it and he couldn't get enough of it. Of course it didn't take me long to figure out the magic ingredient—cilantro! *—Jenny*

Every couple of hours I turn into Satan if I don't eat something.

—Jessica Alba

The Knocked-Up Night Life: Happy Hour for the Pregnant Chick

What's a chick to do when she's got a 40-week pregnant pause in her usual Friday night happy-hour plans? Whatever you do, don't fall into the "bored on baby" syndrome—sitting home while your girls go out without you. After all, happy is more than an hour, and cocktail parties without cocktails are still parties—just reframe your notion of bellying up. Use your "on the wagon" status to encourage your girlfriends to join you in some new adventures.

• Start a new "Mommy and Tea" tradition at an herbal tea café or lure the ladies' night out crowd to chocolate tastings or gourmet cooking classes, or extend the happy hour by taking in a new movie every week, a yoga class, or a pedicure appointment.

• Lobby for some "pregnant party girl" rules such as boycotting establishments with long lines, standing room only, smoking, or a plethora of drunk people.

• Game parties are great too because as a non-drinker you have the intellectual upper hand—and delicious virgin drinks will keep you in high spirits. Learn a few favorite recipes so you can instruct bartenders when needed.

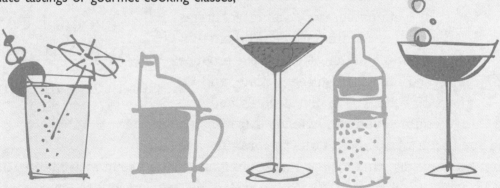

Safe Sex on the Beach

¼ C cranberry juice
¼ C grapefruit juice
¼ C peach nectar

Serve over ice. Garnish with orange slice.

Preggy Piña Colada

¾ C pineapple juice
¼ C coconut cream
1 C crushed ice

Blend ingredients in blender until smooth and frothy. Garnish with pineapple slice.

Manhattan Mama

¼ C cranberry juice
¼ C orange juice
Splash of cherry juice
1 lemon, halved and squeezed

Serve chilled or over ice. Garnish with maraschino cherry.

Nojito

1 sprig of mint
1 lime
1 tsp sugar
1 C club soda

Muddle (crush) the mint, sugar, and juice from the lime using a wooden pestle in the bottom of a shallow glass. Fill the glass with crushed ice. Pour in the club soda and garnish with mint sprig and slice of lime.

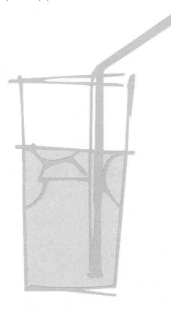

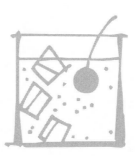

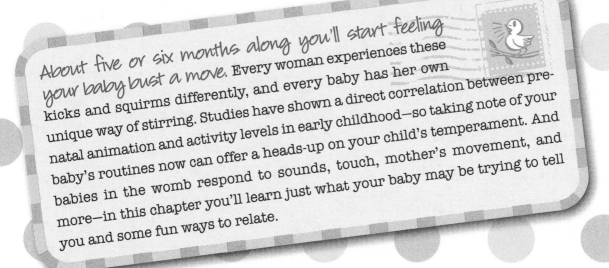

About five or six months along you'll start feeling your baby bust a move. Every woman experiences these kicks and squirms differently, and every baby has her own unique way of stirring. Studies have shown a direct correlation between prenatal animation and activity levels in early childhood—so taking note of your baby's routines now can offer a heads-up on your child's temperament. And babies in the womb respond to sounds, touch, mother's movement, and more—in this chapter you'll learn just what your baby may be trying to tell you and some fun ways to relate.

THE BUMP delivery

IF IT TAKES A VILLAGE, WHY AM I THE ONLY ONE WITH STRETCH MARKS?...

–Ame and Emily

3

3

❀ CHAPTER THREE ❀

3
CHAPTER THREE · CHAPTER THREE · CHAPTER THREE ·

Belly Dancing
Your Bump Gets Busy

Mama Mia: Bjorn Again

When I found out I was pregnant with my first baby, I pored over every baby book I could get my hands on, obsessively charting developmental milestones and researching more on fetal science than most Ph.D. programs require. Early on, I came across the "Mozart effect," and the idea of boosting the IQ of our baby by exposing her to classical music struck a chord. My husband was less than thrilled that his beloved classic rock would be preempted by nine months of classical music. But whenever he bemoaned the loss of Steppenwolf to Wolfgang, I reminded him that Bruce Springsteen was no longer his boss and a little music appreciation could do us all some good. I assured him that when our little Phi Beta Kappa accepted her diploma (Ivy League, of course) he'd realize the sacrifice had been worth it.

My belly swelled along with the soothing strains of sonatas and concertos, and one night as I lay reading in bed my husband removed his headphones to ask, "Do you think she likes it?"

"What?" I replied.

"The music. Do you really think she likes it? What if she's in there going, 'Good grief, woman. Give it a rest!' I mean, how 'bout trying a little CCR or Grateful Dead just to mix things up for her?"

"Show me Jerry Garcia's MENSA card and I'll consider adding him to the playlist. For now, I'm sticking to the real oldies," I replied.

As much as I hated to admit it, his comments nagged at me. What if I *was* imposing music on my baby that she didn't enjoy? Was I already one of *those* moms, so hell-bent on perfection that I'd push my own agenda regardless of how my child felt about it? The thought of giving my baby every advantage I could provide calmed me. Until she could protest, I reasoned, she was at the mercy of my well-intended music choices.

The next night my girlfriends had planned a little field trip to the theater to see the ABBA musical,

Mamma Mia! Up to that point, I'd felt the first stirrings of the baby move—we were past the quickening, fluttery stage but not quite to the really engaging business of big kicks.

My mother told me I was **dancing before I was born.** She could feel my **toes tapping wildly** inside her for months. —*Ginger Rogers*

As we took our seats and the show began, I felt a strong kick for the first time. I excitedly whispered down the row to my friends, who put their hands on my belly, "all-in" style.

"Oooh," we all said in unison as she gave me another stout poke.

About that time, we were blasted by the show's opening medley, to which baby girl gave a succession of even bolder kicks. For the entire musical, my bump was covered by eager hands as we marveled at her enthusiastic response to her introduction to ABBA. "Dancing Queen" was her favorite by far, eliciting a Rockette-worthy performance.

I couldn't wait to get home and tell my husband. Euphoric from finally feeling the baby really kick up her heels, I wasn't even dreading the "I told you so" response he'd rightfully deliver.

"ABBA? Come on," he said instead. But try as I might, I couldn't rouse the baby; she was obviously tired out from her girls' night out.

Come morning, I gave the symphonies an intermission and surprised my husband with a wakeup call of "Take a Chance on Me." The baby kicked in response.

"Okay, now it's my turn," he said, excitedly. He cued up "Sugar Magnolia," and she gave two more big kicks against his eager palm.

"Now *that's* my girl," he said grinning ear to ear as we lay there feeling our little one dance beneath my skin.

❦ Postcard *to the* Bump ❦

The first time I felt you move ....

....

....

....

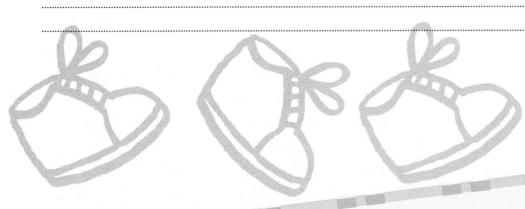

Keeping the Beat I lean against a log and watch a light play in the unfurled oak leaves. Even with my eyes closed I can see the dancer of sun and leaf. Which gives me an idea. I pull down my stretch-panel jeans, roll my shirt up my rib cage, and lie back, belly to the sky. In the sunlight the skin over my abdomen feels taut and tingly. I am a great closed eye-lid. And that's when I feel it for the first time. Like the fluttering of a bird in a cupped hand, only deep inside and down low. –Sandra Steingraber, in "Having Faith: An Ecologist's Journey to Motherhood"

Look Ma, I'm Dancing!

Next to cleavage, belly movements and bumps are one of the most beloved parts of pregnancy and the first tactile connection to our babies. Babies move to get their limbs and muscles ready for the world—and we moms can use their motion as a way to communicate. You might even detect your baby's stirrings in response to noise, food, and your emotions. Later on in your pregnancy you may sense when your baby is asleep or awake. While they can be a wonderful diversion, your baby's movements can also be a source of anxiety as you learn to decipher the rhythm of his or her movements. Your obstetrician will give you the lowdown on what to look for in the realm of fetal movement, and since we fall well into the better-safe-than-sorry camp, listen to her advice and don't hesitate to call if something ever seems amiss.

First Trimester: Though you probably won't feel any real pitter-patters until well into your second trimester, that doesn't mean you can't start touting your baby's first–trimester in utero feats—by the sixth and seventh week of your pregnancy your sweet pea is busy arching and curling his whole body. In the eighth week, he'll be able to move an arm or leg, and by the ninth week your peanut can slowly bring his fingers to his face. By week ten he can even move his little fingers and wave "Hi, Mom!"

After adding the other first trimester accomplishments—hiccupping, stretching, yawning, sucking, swallowing, and grasping—the final tally for a teeny baby is very impressive!

So I am often awake these days in the **hours before the dawn,** full of joy, full of fear. The first birds begin to sing at quarter after five, and when Sam moves around in my stomach, kicking it **feels like there are trout inside of me,** leaping.

—*Anne Lamott,* Operating Instructions

SECOND TRIMESTER: While first steps are still a ways off, during the second trimester your baby's movements will become more obvious and elaborate. She'll exercise her lungs and continue to suck, swallow, and breathe in amniotic fluid. By the fifth month some babies begin sucking their thumbs! During this trimester your baby will also begin to taste, hear, and make facial expressions. With plenty of room to somersault, twist, and turn, she'll engage in some in utero bungee jumping, and you and your partner will applaud every flip and move. Your smart little one will also begin to recognize your voice, flutter her eyelids, and practice grabbing. All this commotion motion adds up to a stellar trimester of accomplishments.

THIRD TRIMESTER: With space getting tighter, your baby's movements might begin to make you more uncomfortable. During this trimester your little one will have detectable waking and resting periods. He can now open his eyes and will even respond to a bright light directed at your stomach. Your baby can inhale and exhale, turn toward noises, and, as sad as it sounds, cry. Your baby Einstein is now in great shape to deal with life on the other side!

Ice Ice Baby!

When I was pregnant with my first baby, I used to freak out about him not moving as much as I wanted, so I would drink TONS of ice water to make him cold and move. I used to joke that he would end up being an artic swimmer. My little guy doesn't seem to need me to throw any water on him now, as he was doing plank and downward dog at four months and was crawling at seven months, so I guess he's pretty physically advanced. Never thought I'd be a stage mother before he was born! —Jill

How Busy Is Your Baby?

Perhaps you'll find your jumping bean in one or more of the descriptions below—or then again you might need to write your own!

THE SNUGGLER. This peewee couch potato is definitely not known for perpetual pounds and kicks on the womb door and moves just enough to keep you from calling 911. But by being passive, your coy little spud is making you pay very close attention to her. We think these little drama queens relish the singular focus on every move they make.

THE POKER. Just when you've finally found a comfortable position on the couch, this little devil jabs you right in the ribs. You'll spend a lot of time pondering just which side of the family those pointy limbs came from (Dad's!) or wondering how your baby managed to gain access to a sharp stick in utero. The sleepless nights, painful punches, and rib-cracking pokes will earn you some internal battle scars as well as bragging rights with the other moms.

THE FIDDLER. Unlike the poker, this gentler little baby seems to be constantly fiddling with his fingers and toes.

One moment you'll think he's trying to carefully dig his way out of there, and the next you'll swear he's drawing stick figures on his womb wall. Piano prodigy? Knitting expert? Writer? Have fun daydreaming about where this finely tuned little tickler's talents will take him—and how proud you'll be!

THE PUZZLER. This baby will really keep you guessing with acrobatic contortions that prove she can be in two places at once. Just when you're certain you've identified two little feet under your right rib cage, a third seems to materialize instantly under your left. These enigmatic kicks and punches make you a walking source of entertainment—if you're willing to share the antics of your little Houdini with an audience.

THE HEAD BANGER. A nonstop moving machine, this baby can get a rise out of even the most seasoned obstetrician and delight his future siblings with hours of fascinating spectacle as he stretches the limits of your skin. Be prepared—as very soon there won't be anything holding back this poster child for baby-proofing.

🥿 Postcard *to the* Bump 🥿

Your style of movement was ....

....

....

A mother's joy begins when
new life is stirring inside, when a
tiny heartbeat is heard for the
very first time, and a playful
kick reminds her that
she is never alone. —*Anonymous*

Mom Always Said . . .

For generations mothers have regaled family members and friends with stories of their babies' in utero activity or, in some cases, plain laziness, with a wink and nod and an "I-told-you-so" tone as they watch their children's corresponding activity outside of the womb. Any time junior lies couch-potato prone or soars Olympics-style over a fence, we moms reassure ourselves that we knew it all along. It wasn't until recently, however, that the medical community decided to find out if mama's theory of relative activity was based on reality or merely a quest to be "right." After studying prenatal activity at 24, 30, and 36 weeks' gestation and comparing that with the activity level of those same babies at one and two years of age, scientists determined that there is a link. In other words, babies who were very active in the womb were very active after they were born, and vice versa. But scientists went even further than Mom and, using advanced ultrasound technology that studied all fetal movement, found that everything a baby does in the womb extends to their outside life, including scowling, smiling, thumb-sucking, and even raising eyebrows and winking!

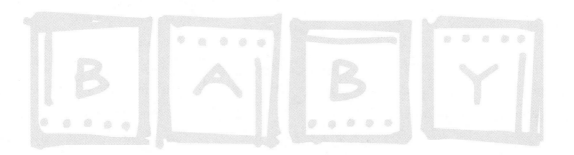

BELLY SHOTS: ULTRA-COOL ULTRASOUND PHOTO PROJECTS

While frames and wallets are fine for most family photos, we think the very first pictures of your little bump deserve ultra-special attention. Create an adorable page in your "While We Were Waiting for You" journal, p. 28, or simply frame and display these fun creations in your precious little egg's nursery.

MOMMY MATTE

Dress in a close-fitting black top and leggings. Pose against a blank wall or light-colored background and have someone take a photo of you from the side to create a shot in silhouette. Print the image to the size you want. Paste a cropped circular photo of baby's ultrasound on your belly before framing.

Search books, magazines, or online for a photo of a nest filled with eggs. Use a scanner or color photocopier to enlarge the image to the size you want, or print out the online photo. Copy your ultrasounds and, using the size of the eggs in the photo as a guide, cut your photos into egg shapes to fill the nest before framing.

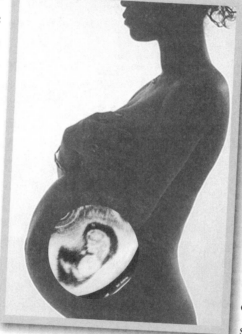

WELCOME MATTE

Frame your baby's ultrasound photo in an oversized, light-colored photo matte. Have family and friends sign it and collect cards, e-mail messages, and letters of congratulations to decoupage or add to the matte, surrounding your baby's first picture in words of love and sweet anticipation. If your bump has siblings, matte a copy of an ultrasound photo and let big brother or sister create a work of art for the baby's nursery using stickers, markers, or crayons.

⚸ Postcard *to the* Bump ⚸

The first time I saw you on the ultrasound I felt ....
....
....
....
....

Happiness pulses
with every beat of my heart.

—*Emily Logan Decens*

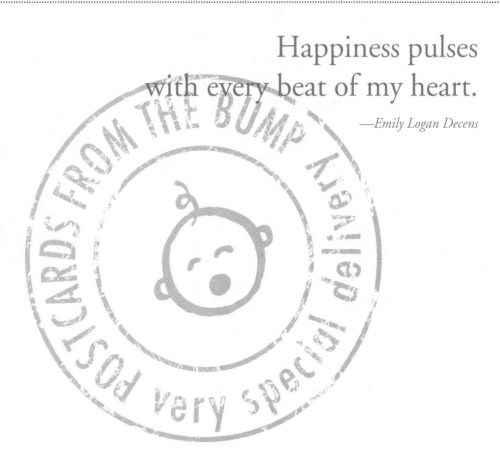

Thumbs Up From my nineteenth week of pregnancy, I knew exactly what my daughter, Ashton, would look like. My husband and I were at our first ultrasound when the technician switched on the monitor and our little girl lit up the screen, perfectly profiled with her right thumb in her mouth and a tiny index finger curled gracefully over the top of her nose. Little did I know how very familiar this black and white image would become to us. Due to some concerns, my doctors ordered ultrasounds every three weeks, and every single time we were greeted by the same adorable pose from our little "Peanut"—right thumb in mouth with the index finger draped over her nose. When Ashton arrived at 37 weeks it was surreal to find myself holding the flesh-and-blood version of that familiar image. Like that scene in *The Wizard of Oz* when the black-and-white world blooms into Technicolor, I cradled in my arms the rose bud–tinted, downy-soft–skinned reality of those ultrasound pictures. Ashton is a second-grader now, and when I peek in on her at night I still find her in that signature pose. And while it may bring about braces and all matter of orthodontia, this is my girl, and I wouldn't change her for the world! —*Jessica*

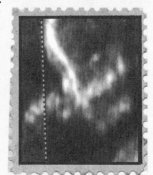

Life is magic, the way nature works
seems to be quite magical.

—*Jonas Salk*

IT TAKES TWO TO TANGO:
Party in My Womb

Ultrasounds give us a bird's-eye view into life on the inside, and some studies of ultrasound activity have shown that twins interact and actually seem to "play" with each other in the womb. During ultrasounds taken during midpregnancy, identical twins have been observed "holding hands," cuddling, and even shoving each other—interactions that persist after birth. Fraternal twins have also been seen "playing" together in utero through the membranes that divide them. In one study, a set of twins, a brother and sister, seemed especially fond of being cheek-to-cheek and developed certain gestures and repetitive movements in relationship to one another in their mother's womb. Later, as toddlers, these same siblings had a favorite game that involved standing on either side of a curtain and poking and tickling each other through the fabric—bearing an uncanny resemblance to the "games" they'd played in utero.

Brotherly Love When I was pregnant with my twins, Benny and Tomås, they gave me some pretty solid clues to their personalities. Benny was our active kicker, and his poor brother and I were, and continue to be, on the receiving end of his rambunctious legs. He needs about half as much sleep as Tomås, who before birth, and still is, my peaceful, sleep-loving little man. Benny followed Tomås around in the womb, always cuddling up to him, which gave my bump an interesting, off-kilter shape since Benny kept Tomås cornered on my left side for the entire pregnancy. To this day Benny is lost without his brother. Tomås loves to eat and was significantly bigger than Ben at birth—I swear he was hogging all the food in utero! We craved fruit when I was pregnant, and it's still their favorite food. —*Nancy*

POSTCARD from the BUMP · POSTCARD from the BUMP

❧ Postcard *to the* Bump ❧

You really got busy when ....
....

....

....

....

....

It goes without saying that you **should never** have more children than you **have car windows.**

—*Erma Bombeck*

My first son used to kick me in one certain spot all the time during my pregnancy. To this day I have a stretch mark in that spot. As it turned out, my "little kicker" became the place kicker on his football team in high school and during his senior year the team went 12-1 (the best record that we had ever had). The big rival was Cullman High (we only beat them about once every 20 years), and we won the game by one point—with the extra point my son managed to kick for the team. After he graduated from high school he walked on the football team at the University of Alabama as a kicker. —Patricia

An Affair to Remember

There was only one word to describe how I felt in my seventh month of pregnancy: "dumpy." I wasn't one of those chicks with a little basketball pregnancy. Far from it. I was a giant amoeba—seemingly boundless and shapeless. But as hard as it was to be a gigantopregnasaurus, losing the attention of my husband at the same time was a bitter prenatal pill to swallow.

Just about the time our baby started to move energetically in my belly, my husband began to act differently. He seemed distant, yet euphoric—too quick to giggle: "Don't you just love to hear little kids laughing?"; too solicitous: "I'll take out the trash."; and too expectant: "Let's go look at strollers today!" While I felt as if I deserved a medal—or a large frosted brownie— every time I walked more than 50 yards, he seemed to have the energy of a five-year-old and the giddiness of someone who had just fallen in love. He was obsessed, distracted, dreamy. He'd get lost in thought every time I tried to discuss anything practical, like what we were going to eat for dinner. It wasn't until my eighth month that I began to suspect he was seeing someone on the side while I snored loudly between trips to the bathroom.

All my suspicions came to a head the day we were supposed to go out for ice cream, and he went AWOL. My desperate calls to his cell phone went straight to voicemail. When he finally came home, long after I had dug out a pint of permafrosted Rocky Road, I confronted him. "Where were you?" I yelled with my hand firmly on the spot that used to be my hip. He stammered and his face reddened, clearly realizing the jig was up. "Babys 'R' Us. I wanted to try out some of the video baby monitors." And there it was. His new little someone had been right under my nose the whole time. And those nightly trysts were happening in my own bed as I slept, with the baby moving vigorously against his back or under his hand.

"The baby and I were playing again last night," he'd coo sleepily in the morning. "Why didn't you wake me up?" I'd ask a little resentfully.

"You needed your rest," he'd respond magnanimously.

Even though I knew I was being absurd—this was his baby, too—the whole thing made me a little crazy. As the mother I felt as if I owned those nine months. I was like the telephone operator who should be asked to connect the call. Bypassing me was just plain disrespectful. There he was, svelte and energetic as always, getting all the benefits without suffering any of the consequences—what did *he* know about swollen ankles, food revulsions, or bras that tightened like barbed-wire corsets with every week that rolled by?

"Maybe your problem isn't with their relationship, it's with yours," counseled my close friend.

"You need more attention and reassurance. Go out together more and try to reconnect."

With very little time left, I scheduled as many date nights as I could to guarantee the one-on-one time I so clearly deserved—I mean, needed.

Our dates began at fancy restaurants with white tablecloths and quiet music—places we knew we wouldn't be eating at after the price of a babysitter was added to the check. We went to old haunts, where I'd teeter on groaning bar stools sipping soda and lime while he nursed a pint and played my favorite songs on the jukebox. Eventually I began to relax with the realization that, come what may, we'd always be a couple. We were eating pizza at the park, watching families swing and play at twilight when I felt the first contraction, and later that night our healthy baby girl was born.

Seeing my husband in action as a father moved me to tears with how gingerly and sweetly he cuddled our daughter. And when I was able to nap while he expertly fed and swaddled our baby, I was extremely grateful for his natural connection to our little girl. As for my own impatience and jealousy, I don't blame myself for feeling that way—coming to terms with motherhood brings a whole host of baffling emotions that need to be sorted, accepted, and laid bare before you can fully embrace it. Threesomes and changes in family makeup, no matter how eagerly anticipated, can be difficult. Maybe I came to it a little slower than some, but I did learn that if you factor in a lot of love, some patience, and a little gratitude, it will always add up to the perfect number.

👟 Postcard *to the* Bump 👟

While we were waiting for you, your Dad and I connected over ....

....

....

....

....

....

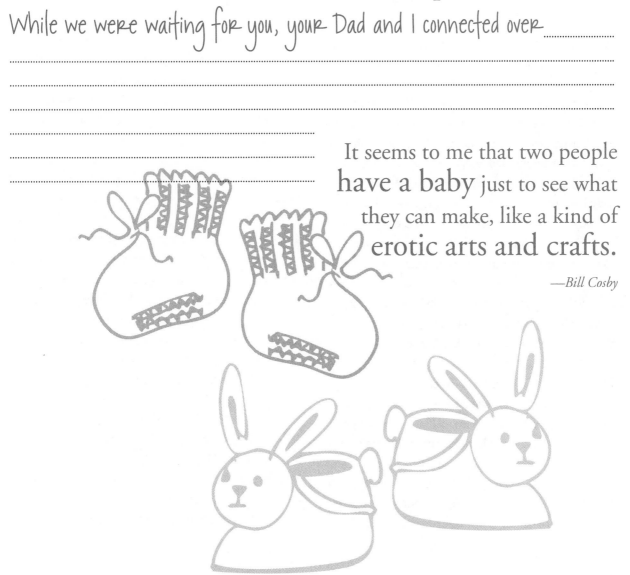

It seems to me that two people
have a baby just to see what
they can make, like a kind of
erotic arts and crafts.

—Bill Cosby

Who's Your Daddy?

Every expectant father handles pregnancy with his own personal flair and, shall we say, rather unique reactions to the reality of impending fatherhood. While we mamas lay claim to the majority of pregnancy symptoms and life-altering experiences, Daddy is dealing with his own host of emotions and world-rocking changes, too. Does this mean he won't ever get to go skydiving? What will happen to his Friday night poker games with the boys? Will he ever get some quality time with you again? Though no one can claim he's dealing with *more than you,* he might require some extra reassurance, handholding, and patience in the months ahead. Here are some tongue-in-cheek descriptions of expectant daddy types (yes, we feel your pain) to help you laugh at their sometimes confounding behavior.

DENIAL DUDE. Instead of registering for baby items, Denial Dude thinks you should catch a matinee, and the only baby face he seems to be interested in is the one on his iPod playlist. He's baffled as to why you don't want to go to a hip-hop concert in week 39 of your pregnancy, and he thinks it's very inconvenient that he has to move his golf clubs out of the backseat to set up the infant carrier. Feeling contractions? He takes a long shower and makes himself a sandwich while you call the doctor and strum your fingers waiting for him to get ready. Good thing you're not spiders—you'd go black widow all over the situation; but before you pinch his head off, realize your inscrutable mate does care deeply. He's just completely terrified. Try to involve him as much as possible by getting him to accompany you to your obstetrician appointments and reading pregnancy books aloud. With a little patience, he'll come around to his sweet new reality in his own sweet time.

THE HE-MAMA. This overly empathetic hubby exhibits more pregnancy symptoms than you do. You feel tired, and he just has to take a nap. You crave chocolate-covered doughnuts, and he inhales two on the way home from the doughnut shop; so it's no wonder he's tipping the scales with a little papa paunch of his own. He's been feeling a little run down, so suddenly he's joining you in taking supplements and guzzling nutritious smoothies. Your feet and back ache, and guess what? His do, too! If you didn't love him so much you'd ask the doctor to prescribe some labor-simulating drugs you could slip into his yo-mamma yogurt while he's checking his ankles for swelling. Ultimately your He-Mama just needs some TLC. Consider it mommy boot camp—and baby him when you can.

Let her have the babies; but after that, try to share every job around. Any man to-day who returns from work, sinks into a chair, and calls for his pipe is a man with an appetite for danger.

—*Bill Cosby*

SOY BOY. This au natural man is apt to go daddy dearest on you if he catches you eating anything from a plastic container or food from a drive-thru. He insists that everything you eat—oh, precious baby vessel—be certified organic, dye-free, nongenetically altered, and of course nutritious. He's your own personal food taster and lives in utter fear that a transfat, food additive, or growth hormone will somehow sneak onto your plate. He constantly fuels his paranoia with Internet and newsmagazine "research," and you've even caught him writing down the ingredients in your hair conditioner. If you're dying to consume some French fries or nachos (and what pregnant woman isn't?) tell no one and destroy all evidence of your transgression.

SUPER STUD. His sperm is bigger, faster, and stronger than any other daddy—able to circumvent diaphragms in a single bound, bust through spermicidal foam like a speeding bullet, and swim the backstroke in record time. Your pregnancy might have been a surprise to you, but your Man of Steel's confidence in his ability to procreate was beyond reproach. Infertility? He's never heard of it. Although your pregnancy might have boosted his prowess permanently, he'll still need support to make the leap to fatherhood, where he'll join the ranks of real men who change diapers, warm bottles, and sing lullabies. Fear not—he's bound to be a Super Daddy.

DR. DADDY. You never knew you married an OB/GYN until you got pregnant. Suddenly your handsome number-one doctor is regaling you with pregnancy facts and studies. Did you know your blood flow has increased by 40 percent? Or what to look for during an ultrasound? Not to worry, he's read your chart and knows all the vitals. He's more present at your doctor visits than you are and is always armed with a notepad of thoughtful questions. Before you hit the delivery room, be sure to remind him to set aside the physician robes, as it's time for him to play mere old Daddy.

From Beer to Paternity: Making a Pop Star

Somewhere between your twentieth and twenty-fifth week of pregnancy is the ideal time to help your aspiring Daddy-O become even more comfortable with the bump. Your baby's ability to move, hear, and taste presents a variety of ways for Dad to start to relate to his baby, and a little interaction now will go a long way in boosting his confidence before the big birth day actually arrives.

IN A DEEP VOICE. Studies such as "The Cat in the Hat Study" have shown that newborns do recognize the voices of their family members when they're born, and Daddy's deeper voice is sure to resonate with your little one. Perhaps Dad could begin a bedtime ritual for the bump, such as reading a story with a catchy cadence that the bump can groove to. Or if he's more of a crooner than a reader, he can hum a melody, part of a song he loves, or simply play a favorite tune from his playlist for a lullaby. Science has proven that it is possible for babies to remember songs, books, and voices they heard repeatedly before birth, so give your baby a paternal preview.

TOUCH FOOTBALL. Bearing the bump has its benefits—like being the first to feel your baby move—but those womb workouts are also an ideal opportunity for your partner to get in on the fun. For most pregnant mothers, your little bun gets busy just as you lay down at night, and begins to be detectable sometime after your twentieth week. Invite Daddy to participate in the action by first holding his hand to the spots where your baby can be felt. The more touching and stroking Baby Daddy does, the more likely he is to really connect with the bump.

SUGAR DADDY. By your sixth or seventh month of pregnancy you might have noticed your baby's response to certain foods—particularly sweets. Encourage Daddy to mix you up a Coco-Bean Smoothie (p. 105) or feed you some Goo-goo Ga-ga Cookies (p. 55). He can serve you while telling his little one that these sweet treats are "from Daddy with love." Reassure him that you're just being completely selfless here.

❧ Postcard *to the* Bump ❧

The sweetest thing your Dad did while we were pregnant was ....

....

....

....

....

....

....

My father used to play with **my brother and me** in the yard. Mother would come out and say, "You're tearing up the grass." **"We're not raising grass,"** Dad would reply. "We're raising boys."

—*Harmon Killebrew*

☙ Postcard *to the* Bump ☙

Your Dad loved to read/sing
....
....
....
....
....

When I was six months pregnant with my baby girl, my son, Jared (two years old), was mesmerized by the movements of my belly. He got very excited and said, "Mommy, the baby touched me . . . I need to turn it off." He then pointed the remote control to Mommy's tummy. If only we had known how many times we would wish that was an option once Annelise was born! —Andria

Stripes or Solid Sean, my husband, often missed out on our baby's movements. As we'd lie in bed reading or watching TV and I'd feel her move I'd shout, "Sean, put your hand on my belly!" But she always seemed to take a break the minute Sean put his hand on the right spot. It made me feel bad that he couldn't feel her like I could, as her movements were really magical. That Fourth of July I opted to wear a navy-and red-striped shirt over a solid red tee. I told Sean to watch my belly throughout the day. "When the lines arch and shift, the baby is changing position." He didn't seem to think it was such a big deal until he saw it himself. I'm not sure if he felt too much of an emotional connection until that moment. I knew that he took pride in his "accomplishment" because of the copious Blackberry notes he took at the prenatal visits, breastfeeding classes, and birthing seminars. But I think that the reality that I was carrying a person inside of me didn't ring true to him until she began to dance.
I wonder how Baby Nora will like wearing stripes. —Bridget

All the time we **wondered and wondered,** who is this person coming/growing/turning/floating/swimming **deep, deep inside.**

—*Crescent Dragonwagon*

Dressed to the Nine Months

Most of us self-sacrificing types (we *are* mothers, after all) tend to put our own needs aside for our offspring, but even if you're the kind of chick who would return something at Baby Gap and use the credit on the "Mama" side of the store, you probably don't want to drop too much coin on clothes you can wear only for a few months. Here are some tips from knocked-up knockouts, a.k.a. pregnant fashionistas, who, though they don't regularly, if ever, pose for *Vogue*, do walk the walk when it comes to the latest in bumpwear.

JEANS: Don't let anything come between you and a great pair of jeans, not even your bump. Invest in a high-quality pair of maternity jeans in a current cut that flatters your blossoming figure. Take the time to find a great fit. This wardrobe staple can be dressed up or down—for a night out or a visit to your prospective pediatrician.

SHOES: A comfy yet flattering shoe is de rigueur for the pregnant chick. If you can tolerate a sturdy heel, the height will give you a leaner look and visually extend your legs. Save the stilettos for après bump unless you're a seasoned runway model—they can give you backaches and wreak havoc on your center of gravity. While at the end of your pregnancy you might be forced to don a pair of flip-flops, but a cute pair of sandals or boots will give you some fashion flair for most of your nine months.

CRISP WHITE BLOUSE AND BLACK PANTS: Think Katharine Hepburn with a bump. A classic white blouse with a stylish collar and cuffs paired with a sweeping pair of black pants will take you anywhere. A string of pearls and you're off to the opera; funky bangles and you're ready for Pearl Jam.

TUBE SKIRTS: These wonderful little inventions are comfortable, versatile, and fashionable. They also have the remarkable ability to stretch beyond your wildest nightmares—oops . . . we mean dreams! In winter pair one with tights and cozy boots, for summer add a tee shirt and sandals—they do everything but wash themselves.

ACCESSORIES: As rah-rah as we are about pregnancy, even we have to admit that at a certain point you will be sick to death of your clothes and ready to move out of the pregnancy rack entirely. That's when you turn your attentions to the sweet little things in the accessories aisle—sunglasses, jewelry, maybe a chic handbag, a shade hat, or cute scarves—anything that gives you the boost you need to get through those final weeks. Think of it as a fashion epidural—a little shot of distraction to take the edge off.

WHAT TO AVOID: No matter how great Gwyneth might look in sleeveless pregnancy tanks, avoid them, as well as horizontal fabric patterns, shapeless dresses, and robe-style voluminous sweaters. And please leave the overalls to the farmers—you'll look like you're trying to steal a watermelon.

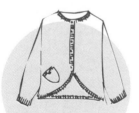

Fashion can be bought.
Style one must possess.

—*Edna W. Chase*

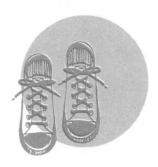

⚓ Postcard *to the* Bump ⚓

When I was pregnant with you, I treated myself to

A Mother Hen Told Us... Jewelry—
be it costume or fine—is an excellent "investment" during pregnancy. A well-chosen piece of jewelry can make the most inexpensive outfit look like a million bucks. The best part? Always a perfect fit.

GET IT OFF YOUR CHEST, BABY: NO BORING BIBS

You'll soon realize that no matter how darling you outfit your precious little doll, her carefully chosen ensembles will spend a lot of time hidden (and protected) behind a bib. Spit happens, but there are fun and fashionable ways to address it. While you're waiting for that bump to bake, make up a stash of tongue-in-cheek bibs so your little mess can spill it with style. You can purchase blank bibs and printable iron-on transfer paper from craft stores and online. Believe it or not, junior can dirty as many as four a day. Have fun putting words in your baby's mouth!

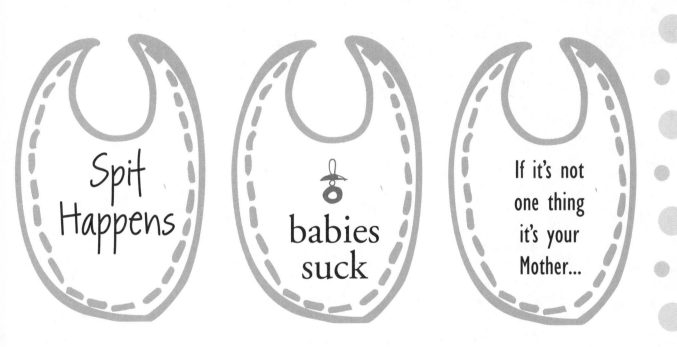

Spit Happens

babies suck

If it's not one thing it's your Mother...

Laughing on the Inside My five-year old daughter, Claire, has by all accounts one of the best giggles I've ever heard. Since about the age of two, she ends a giggle fit with a long sigh and one of two trademark phrases, "oooooh, you crack me out" or "oooooh, I crack me out." While my older daughter never had the hiccups in utero, Claire had them constantly. So, I'm left to ponder if maybe Claire was "cracking herself out" from the beginning! —Ellen

U.S. POSTAGE

HEAVEN SENT

Little creature, formed for joy and mirth.—*William Blake*

Smoothie Talking Mama

When you're carrying a bump it's the perfect time to become a smoothie talking mama. Here are some satisifying smoothies to try.

Ju-Ju Berry

1 C strawberries, halved with stems removed
½ banana, sliced
1 C vanilla yogurt
4–5 ice cubes
¼ C orange juice

Blend all ingredients in blender until smooth.

Razzberry

1 C frozen raspberries
¾ C vanilla frozen yogurt
½ C vanilla soy milk
⅛ tsp almond extract
1 tsp honey

Blend all ingredients in blender until smooth.

Coco-Bean

1 C chocolate yogurt
½ C vanilla yogurt
1 T chocolate sauce
½ C milk
4–5 ice cubes

Blend all ingredients in blender until smooth.

Little Pumpkin

1 C vanilla soy milk
1 medium banana, sliced
¼ C canned pumpkin
1 dash cinnamon
2 T maple syrup
4 ice cubes

Blend all ingredients in blender until smooth.

Blueberries for the Bump

½ banana
1 C blueberries
1 C lemon yogurt
¼ C grape juice
1 tsp honey

Blend all ingredients in blender until smooth.

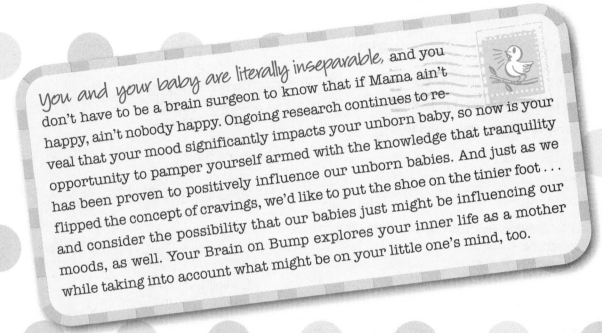

You and your baby are literally inseparable, and you don't have to be a brain surgeon to know that if Mama ain't happy, ain't nobody happy. Ongoing research continues to reveal that your mood significantly impacts your unborn baby, so now is your opportunity to pamper yourself armed with the knowledge that tranquility has been proven to positively influence our unborn babies. And just as we flipped the concept of cravings, we'd like to put the shoe on the tinier foot . . . and consider the possibility that our babies just might be influencing our moods, as well. Your Brain on Bump explores your inner life as a mother while taking into account what might be on your little one's mind, too.

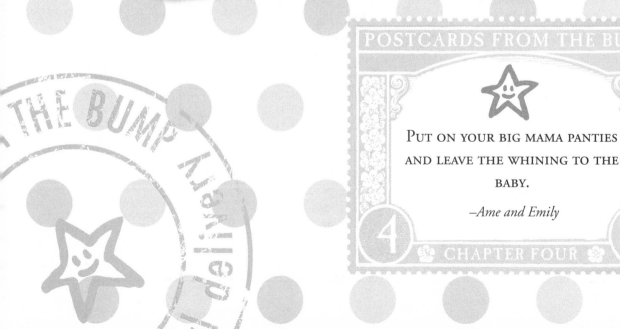

POSTCARDS FROM THE BUMP

PUT ON YOUR BIG MAMA PANTIES
AND LEAVE THE WHINING TO THE
BABY.

–Ame and Emily

4   CHAPTER FOUR   4

CHAPTER FOUR

4

Your Brain on Bump

Moods, Memories, and Dreams of the Pregnant Chick

Funny Baby My firstborn showed himself to me in a dream when I was only a few months pregnant. In the dream, he was about two years old, standing in my sister's bedroom in our childhood home, and he was laughing and laughing, in a way that made me feel giddy and delighted.

I remember thinking that maybe this meant if I had a boy, it would be all right; we would still connect with each other. But how could I, a girly-girl, have a boy? Despite this dream, I remained convinced I'd have a girl, whom we would call Melissa. We had a boy. The first of three. And his middle name is Isaac, after my grandfather. It turns out that Isaac means "laughter" in Hebrew. And laughter is still the way that we connect—18 years later. —Susan

Laughter is the shortest distance
between two people.

—*Victor Borge*

Nine Months of World Domination

As soon as I began to show, I realized that my bump had the uncanny ability to provoke the inner advice columnist, amateur therapist, and recreational OB/GYN in most everyone I met. People who, months before, would have had nothing to say to me were suddenly struck, savant-like, at the sight of my big belly. Everyone wanted to share the most intimate details of their lives or give me overbearing, specific instructions. It was as if their unique brand of maternity genius had lain dormant waiting for the perfect catalyst to unlock it—a pregnant woman waddling down aisle five looking for graham crackers and mini-marshmallows.

Sometimes these encounters were incredibly sweet, like the time a grandmother in a yellow leisure suit and enormous pearl earrings stood patting my hand as she reminisced about the awe she felt when her first baby moved inside her. Another time a harried mother of three, who grabbed at her kids while steadying toppling items from shelves, stood transfixed amid her chaos when she saw my bump. She smiled knowingly at my midsection before locking eyes with me in a moment of motherly solidarity. I wished she'd had the time to elaborate on whatever it was behind that wise smile. At the coffee shop a distinguished older man in an elegant gray suit respectfully asked if he could place his hand on my belly—he'd recently found out that his only daughter was expecting his first grandchild. As he reverently came into contact with my bump, she surprised him with a little kick. "Showoff," I said, and we both laughed.

Moments like these made me feel like a rotund Zen temple—a fertile goodwill ambassador with a plump Buddha belly radiating hope and promise. I was a big hunk of Blarney stone, and I felt generous, bountiful, and elated by what I could so easily share with the world.

Then there were the other times. The checkout clerk who regaled me between register beeps with the excruciating details of her 56-hour "back" labor that ended in an emergency C-section. I managed

There is no delight in owning anything unshared.

—Seneca

to juggle my bags and escape, just as she was lifting her monogrammed smock to show me the scar. And then there were the "doctors" who left me puzzling as to when they'd found time to attend medical school *and* run a dry-cleaning business, roll sushi, manage a Starbucks, sell shoes, or volunteer at the elementary school. One day when my ankles were a tad swollen, a woman practically tried to kidnap me and rush me to the ER in her frantic certainty that I had severe preeclampsia. I headed straight to my real doctor, who confirmed mild edema, then prescribed elevating my feet as well as my water intake and lectured me on the dangers of talking to strangers.

I am a talk-to-strangers, you-show-me-yours-and-I'll-show-you-mine type of chick, but pregnancy challenged even my social tolerances. I had my limits: No touching without asking, and never by weirdos. If questions became too personal I feigned an immediate need for a bathroom and excused myself. And I *never* told strangers the real names we were considering—really, who needs a seed of doubt planted by someone you'll never see again?

My mother always said that all bets are off in respect to privacy when you're pregnant—the whole world knows what you've been doing, and when that baby's ready to come you won't care who sees your lady parts. The same hormones that had me crying at phone commercials and cursing Ben & Jerry's for not making ice cream in five gallon-sized buckets, laid me bare to people's efforts to seek communion with my bump. And really—who could blame them for wanting in on my miracle?

Deep down inside, I suppose I selfishly hope that the goodwill will karmically boomerang back one day when I find myself old and wearing my own leisure suit. I like to think my future holds a kind stranger who, recognizing my wish to revisit the miracle that had happened to me so many years ago, will bless me with an invitation to rest my hand upon her ripe belly.

☆ Postcard *to the* Bump ☆

When people wanted to touch you I felt ....
....
....
....
....

Just Peachy Since my husband always calls me Peach, we christened our first bump Pit. . . . The next time we had twins, we called them the Buds, as in "flower buds" or "little buddies." No matter how old they get or how tall they grow, our children will always be our little "Pit" and "the Buds." —Colleen

Cute as a Button?

O h," my husband said one morning as I stood before the full-length mirror inspecting my enormous 8½-month pregnant belly. His mouth remained frozen in an *O*, his brows knit together, emphasizing his next words: "I didn't know a belly button could *do* that."

Neither did I. And it was *my* belly button. The very same belly button that I'd had all my life, the one that had remained boring, steadfast, and pretty much true to form throughout my last pregnancy. I didn't recognize this freaky in-your-face version of my formerly shy innie. My midsection called to mind the crudely knotted end of a very, very big balloon, and the worst part was the color—my belly button was a bizarre shade of pinky-purple, reminiscent of a fresh bruise with white stretch marks bisecting it west to east.

"You look like you're going to pop," my husband said as he took a few steps back.

"If it weren't so hot, I'd wrap the whole thing in bubble wrap," I replied.

It was the middle of summer, and tissue-thin cotton felt stifling, so I couldn't even wear bulky clothing to disguise my odd little appendage. Whenever I ate in public, well-intended strangers would discreetly point out that something had fallen down my décolletage and migrated south to my belly.

"You dropped a piece of popcorn down your shirt, honey," a nice lady said at the movie theater. "Thank you," I replied, pretending to brush it away as I hurried off before she could see the "popcorn" wasn't going anywhere.

One day, as I put away some laundry in my daughter's dresser, a small collection of pinch pots she'd made in art camp caught my eye. With its muddied glaze of rosy lilac and crimped edges, one bore a striking resemblance to my new, bump–altered belly button. I'd always told her that the little pinkish pot was my favorite and that it reminded me of a rose. Ergo, if the pinch pot looked like a rose (and my belly button looked like the pinch pot), then my belly button could be reinterpreted as a rose—a vast improvement from the knotted latex or the stray snack foods that I'd been comparing it to. And in the vein of the Chinese proverb "There is only one pretty child in the world, and every mother has it," I began to appreciate my unique little "pinch pot."

My belly button didn't look like anyone else's, but that was the beauty of it—like the baby beneath it, it was a fingerprint of creation that could never be imitated. I contemplated it in a whole new light those last weeks of pregnancy, even showing it off to friends, who all echoed my husband's puzzled, slightly bewildered "Oh." "Isn't it cool?" I'd ask. Everyone had to agree they'd never seen anything quite like it.

My son was born on a sweltering, thunderstorm-laden day, and as the

Everything has beauty,
but not everyone sees it.

—Confucius

doctors cut the cord to separate us, the same feeling washed over me as when my daughter was born, a maternal surge of irony—sorrow tinged with great joy. My little guy's now a toddler, and he has the cutest little belly button you've ever seen—a perfect little innie. Given that he's male, barring some freak accident or gross neglect, he'll be able to keep that cute little belly button all his life. And like all mothers who sacrifice, I take totally undeserved—but extremely gratifying—credit for forfeiting my own for his.

Ignorance Is Bliss:
Bumping the Bad Stuff to the Curb

Pregnancy, with all its excitement and happiness, can also be fraught with nerve-racking firsts, unexpected surprises, and more than its share of anxiety. The best defense is a good offense, so equip yourself with some strategies to cope with bumpy spots like uninvited advances from strangers, TMI from family members, and worst-case scenarios that seem to lurk like scary pop-ups within every book or magazine. We're not saying you should bury your head in the sand; just strive for a healthy balance that helps you focus on the positives, not obsess over the fears.

GET A REALITY CHECK. The odds are overwhelmingly in your favor that both you and your baby will be just fine. The percentages of pregnancies that result in healthy babies and healthy mothers rise steadily, year after year. Take comfort that historically you live in a world of groundbreaking obstetrical science, neonatal medicine, and lifesaving technology. Talk to your doctor about your fears and concerns and ask her about any diagnostic tests that may safely reassure you.

IT'S NATURAL. Pregnancy is a completely natural experience, not a condition to be cured or treated like an ailment. Prenatal care is quite simple—nourishment, healthy foods, rest, and abstaining from substances that could harm your baby. Millions of women have done this successfully before you, as is evident by the existence of a growing, thriving human race.

MAKE THE WORRY WORK. It would be great if you could skip along singing a Bobby McFerrin song (actually, it would be very annoying), but that's, thankfully, not practical. Worry comes with every experience, especially pregnancy, and as much as we don't want to, we all succumb to our anxieties to a degree. If a worry nags you, use it to instigate action and seek information. Once you've investigated and sought counsel from your doctor, let the worry go and concentrate on letting what you've learned empower and comfort you.

PRIVACY, PLEASE. Contrary to what many people believe, pregnancy does *not* make you public property. Attention can be nice, but even the most gregarious of mother hens needs to put up her guard once in a while. Luckily, the same state that draws the focus can be used to divert it. Excuse yourself to the bathroom/doctor's appointment/ fresh air when someone's getting too chatty or personal for your comfort. Deflect people from patting your bump with a simple, "Please don't, it makes me uncomfortable," or beat them to it by putting your hand on your belly. Tired of the same questions over and over? Make yourself a custom tee shirt that answers it all up front: "I'm due in September, it's a girl, I feel great, have a nice day."

CLOSE THE BOOK. Don't get us wrong—we're all for reading—but if you're losing precious sleep from poring over the worrisome sections of pregnancy books, it might be time to turn the page. There's a big difference between educating yourself and traumatizing yourself. You know what to expect when you read certain books, and a good bedtime story is not it—read something uplifting and comforting before you turn out the lights, and save the scary stuff for days when you'll be seeing your doctor and can get her expert opinion on the topic.

FIND A POSITIVE PLAYMATE. Another great way to excise the negatives and get yourself into a better mental headspace is to spend some time with a positive girlfriend. Whether she's pregnant or not, a good gal pal can help you put things in perspective and lighten your mental load. It might be a placebo, but regular time on the phone or in person with a friend is some of the best medicine your obstetrician won't likely prescribe.

You see that little squirrel out there in that tree? **She has babies, and she has never read a book.** Maybe it is not quite that simple, but it is not half as complicated as the books, neighbors, grandparents and doctors would make you think it is.

—*Dr. Leila Denmark*

Dream Baby When I was pregnant with my second baby, I had a recurring dream that I wasn't pregnant. In the dreams, I'd go to bed with my big belly, happy and excited, but when I "woke up" in the morning I'd discover that I hadn't been pregnant after all—that the whole thing had been wishful thinking. Afterward I'd wake up confused and greatly relieved to find that my bump was indeed real. I tried to see the dream for what it was—a harmless, subconscious way of coping with my fears and my disbelief that I was being blessed by getting to have another baby.

That little bump turned out to be a healthy baby boy. He's always been a good sleeper, but once in a while he'll wake up in the middle of the night crying hard—as if he's had a bad dream. Now three, he was finally able to tell me what's been so upsetting—"Mama, you were gone," he said through the tears one night. As I comforted and rocked him, I told him the story of how I used to dream that he was gone, too, but that I always woke up to find him . . . and that I'd be here when he woke up, too. *—Amelia*

Only thing worth stealing is a kiss from a sleeping child.

—*Joe Houldsworth*

If you find yourself a bit prone to welling up with emotion, and if certain types of books leave you stranded in the middle of a giant anxiety attack, it's time to completely adjust your reading list. During pregnancy our surging hormones make it necessary for many of us to avoid anything too sad or upsetting—particularly if it involves children—from now through the postpartum months. Here's a list of "pregnancy-safe" positive reads.

I Capture the Castle by Dodie Smith

Cold Comfort Farm by Stella Gibbons

Lucky Jim by Kingsley Amis

Isabel's Bed by Elinor Lipman

How Elizabeth Barrett Browning Saved My Life by Mameve Medwed

Good in Bed by Jennifer Weiner

Dakota by Kathleen Norris

Good friends, good books and a sleepy conscience; this is the ideal life.

—*Mark Twain*

☆ Postcard *to the* Bump ☆

My favorite book when I was pregnant with you was ....

....

....

....

....

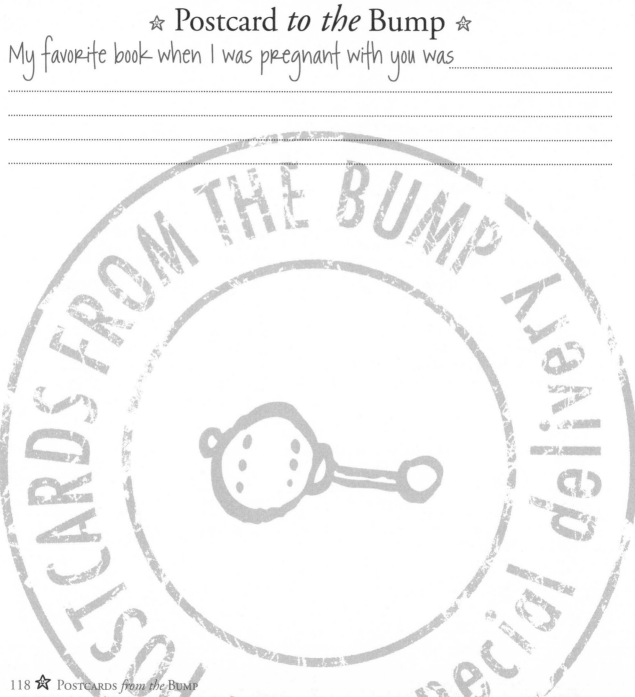

The Name Game

"Have you thought of a name?"

It's the question every expectant parent hears again and again. My husband and I scoured name books and our family tree, and we ran through historically significant monikers, but nothing clicked. Our baby seemed to want nothing to do with choosing a name and gave no inkling of a response—not even a tiny flail or nudge—to any of the many names we threw out.

One night while I dreamed, two words seemed to float into my subconscious from an unseen speaker: "Smedley. Redbone." "Smedley Redbone?" I said after I awoke. Our baby kicked in recognition.

After that we eagerly told friends and family and even the pediatrician our baby's "name." No, Smedley wasn't a permanent name, only a uterine name. At birth "Smedley" was not a boy, as our relatives and several strangers had predicted, but a girl. She relinquished her uterine name gracefully, becoming Risë Amanda in the afterbirth world. Her name reflects the laughter and love that she is. And Smedley Redbone? Retired, but not forgotten. —Beth

Baby Talk

It may be a little while before face-to-face introductions with your little one are possible, but you can boost the heart-to-heart interaction by giving your bump a special little love name. They might be temporary, but in utero "nicknames" help both parents, siblings, and other relatives do some pre–birth day bonding. And besides, who wants to be called "it" for nine months? For inspiration, ponder some nicknames that others have given to the sweet babies in their bellies.

Bean
Boo
Bucket Head
Bud
Buddy Bear
Bun
Bunny
Chimichanga
Chunk
Doll
Egg
Fluff
Hamhock
Junior
Little Bit

Little Dude
Little Fish
Melon
Monkey
Muffin
Munchkin
Nougat
Nut
Peach
Peanut
Petunia
Pit
Pooh
Poppet
Pork Chop

Pudding
Pumpkin
Punk
Rockette
Rooster
Rootie Tootie
Sassafras
Sprout
Sunshine
Sweet Pea
Sweets
Tadpole
Tater
Toot

✯ Postcard *to the* Bump ✯

We called you ....

....

....

....

I have called you by name.
You are mine. —*Isaiah 43:1*

DALAI MAMA:
Find a Happy Place

Not to stress you out, but in addition to eating right, getting plenty of sleep, finding a pediatrician, installing an infant car seat, and scheduling umpteen doctor appointments, did you know that you also need to relax? Yes, it's true. Some studies have indicated that stress can negatively affect your baby. Before you flip out (breathe in, breathe out), let us remind you that most pregnant mothers are just like you, fielding phone calls and running errands, and thousands of healthy babies are born every day. Our take on the "science" is to have fun, be positive, and participate in safe activities that make you, and therefore your bump, happy and healthy. So here are a few tips on how to have peace of mind and practice a little Zen in the art of the mommy-to-be-maintenance.

GET PHYSICAL: Whether it's walking, dancing, swimming, or simply stretching, do some sort of physical activity that's been cleared by your doctor, three to four times a week.

SCHEDULE REGULAR "GIRL TIME": Get together as often as you can with your favorite gal pals. Whether it's on the phone or face-to-face, your girlfriends' support and energy will help you relax, laugh, and set aside your worries.

SCHEDULE A TIMEOUT: Make time for some prebedtime reading, a leisurely evening swim, a Saturday afternoon nap, or just some stolen time lis-

Every pregnant woman should be surrounded with every possible comfort.

—*Dr. Flora L.S. Aldrich*

tening to music. It's important to schedule moments to relax and take it easy every day. If you need to create that special nook to get away from it all and zone out, turn to p. 146 for tips and help.

ASK FOR HELP: Everyone feels good about helping out expectant mothers, so you're really doing others a huge favor by asking them to come to your rescue. Whether it's hanging a picture, changing kitty litter, or taking out the trash, cash in that pregnancy chip so you can conserve your energy for what counts.

STAY POSITIVE: Try not to obsess on negative or anxiety-provoking images or feelings and seek out movies, books, or television shows that up your happy quotient.

SPOIL YOURSELF SILLY: Indulge in things that make you happy—go see a romantic comedy with the father-to-be, get tickets to a much-hyped museum exhibit, buy a beautiful bouquet of flowers, or give yourself permission to loll away an afternoon window shopping with a girlfriend. And do NOT feel guilty about it.

CHANGE IT UP: If there's something in your life such as a volunteer activity or a needy friend that drags you down, now is the time to take a break. You have no better excuse to get out of something than saying that you're "with child" and need your rest. Taking care of you takes care of baby, too.

Hormones on Parade

If you're pregnant no one need remind you of the hormone parade that's marching full-tilt through your body. Perhaps you've blamed those little buggers for your mood swings, weariness, and nausea, but those hormones aren't all bad—they're just trying to keep the rhythm of life steady and strong. Extend a little peace, love, and understanding to your hormones and yourself, and you just might begin to appreciate the tune even if you don't always feel like getting up and dancing.

• **HUMAN CHORIONIC GONADOTROPIN (hCG)** can be thanked for that positive pregnancy test result. The hormone hCG is produced only during pregnancy, and though it heralds the life-changing news, some researchers blame hCG for the morning sickness and fatigue some women experience in the early weeks of pregnancy. Sneak a lunchtime chair massage, an afternoon nap, or a ridiculously early bedtime and blame it on the hCG.

• **PROGESTERONE** is a hardworking hormone whose levels rise as pregnancy progresses. Among other things, it supports placental health, stimulates the growth of breast tissue, and protects the baby by keeping the uterus from contracting. Progesterone can have a calming and soothing effect on an expectant woman's body—in essence, it works with you to help you slow down and relax. Request breakfast in bed, relegate the housecleaning, and put your feet up compliments of progesterone.

• **ESTROGEN,** the definitive chick hormone, works hand-in-glove with progesterone to protect and support your pregnancy from the moment of conception. In a rush of true "girl power," estrogen levels can surge up to a thousand times the amount

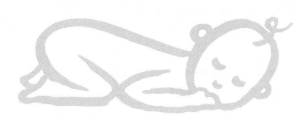

you had in your body before pregnancy. Since it improves blood supply, you can thank estrogen for pumping up everything from cleavage to blood vessels. At the end of your pregnancy, estrogen and progesterone levels lower, and that's when the hormone prolactin, aided by thyroid hormones and insulin, stimulates lactation. You can't beat Mother Nature, so join her by celebrating with a lacy new bra in a bigger size, indulging your appetite for a decadent craving, and treating yourself to an estrogenfest in the form of a girls' night out.

• **OXYTOCIN** as mentioned in Chapter One, is like hitting the hormone jackpot for pregnant mamas. We like to call it, "the happy hormone," since pleasure stimulates its release. Feel-good experiences from orgasm to cuddling to nursing a baby to eating chocolate can stimulate oxytocin. When you hold your newborn in your arms, the oxytocin that triggered your labor and contractions fuels your maternal instincts to nurture and bond with your little one. Jumpstart your endorphins and notch up the oxytocin with pampering pastimes like indulging in a pregnancy massage, baking up a batch of Dark Chocolate Love Bark (p. 27), or doing some serious snuggling on the couch with the one you love.

The Chick Prescription

Your stress level can certainly rise when you're pregnant, and if trying to chill out has you freaking out, consider a landmark study on women's friendships that came out in 2000. The authors of the study, Doctors Shelley Taylor and Laura Klein of UCLA, observed in their lab that when men were stressed they had a tendency to hole up alone, while women would do the opposite—and gather together for coffee. They analyzed the current research on stress and noticed that up until then very little of it included women. Feeling they were onto something, the doctors began to study stress specific to its effects on women. Soon into their study, they discovered that women do indeed tend to respond to stress very differently than men. Instead of the "fight or flight" response to elevated stress, women "tend and befriend" and nurture children or gather with friends. It seems that stress releases oxytocin in women, which encourages us to care for children or spend time with others, and these activities then release even more oxytocin, which further counters stress and produces a calming effect. Additionally, another landmark study—the Nurses Health Study out of Harvard Medical School—found that friendship among women had a profoundly positive impact on their health and longevity and that the more friends women had, the less likely they were to become physically disabled and the more likely they were to lead a happy life. So take heart—and phone a friend!

Suppose you are expecting a child. You need to **breathe and smile** for him or her. Please don't wait until your baby is born before beginning to take care of him or her. You can **take care of your baby right now,** or even sooner. . . . Anything you are, anything you do, is for your baby. . . . Can you tell me that you cannot smile? Think of the baby, and **smile for him, for her,** for the future generations.

—*Thich Nhat Hahn,* Being Peace

☆ Postcard *to the* Bump ☆

When you were my bump, I loved ....

....

....

....

....

....

What the Bump Wants, the Bump Gets Twice as Goods!

As your bump bulges, you may find yourself unable to stomach big meals. You may not be able to pile on the food, but you can pack in some tasty nutrition with little snacks neither you nor your bump will be able to resist.

Preggy Power Bars

1 C raw almonds
¼ C sesame seeds
1½ C quick-cooking oatmeal
½ C dried cranberries
1 C dried blueberries
⅔ C maple syrup
2 T flax seed
1 tsp cinnamon

Preheat oven to 275 degrees. Line a nine-inch baking dish with nonstick aluminum foil.

In a food processor, grind the almonds into a coarse meal. Mix the almonds and the rest of the ingredients in a large bowl.

Using wet fingers, press the mixture into the pan and bake for one hour. Allow to cool in the pan and cut into squares.
Makes about 15 small bars.

Preggy Veggie Dip

2 C small-curd cottage cheese
½ C cream cheese
¼ C scallions, chopped fine
¼ C radishes, chopped fine
2 T chopped fresh parsley
1 T coarsely chopped fresh dill
¼ tsp garlic salt
¼ tsp kosher salt
¼ tsp fresh pepper

Using a hand mixer, mix until smooth. Chill before serving. Makes 3 cups. Serve with vegetables, whole-wheat crackers, pita bread, or pretzels.

Swell Mix

1 C dark chocolate chips
1 C organic dried cherries
1 C vanilla granola

Mix ingredients and store in a covered container or food storage bag.

Mom's the Word

During her first live, on-air audition for the job of cohost for the *Live with Regis and Kathie Lee* show, Kelly Ripa interviewed psychic Char Margolis. During the conversation Margolis shocked everyone, but no one more than Ripa, when she outed the interviewee's little secret on live TV—a bump. The stunned Ripa blushed and confirmed that she was indeed pregnant with her second baby but that she hadn't even told her boss yet. Ripa named her bump Lola, which means "sorrows," but there's nothing sad about how her mom nailed the job—secret bump and all.

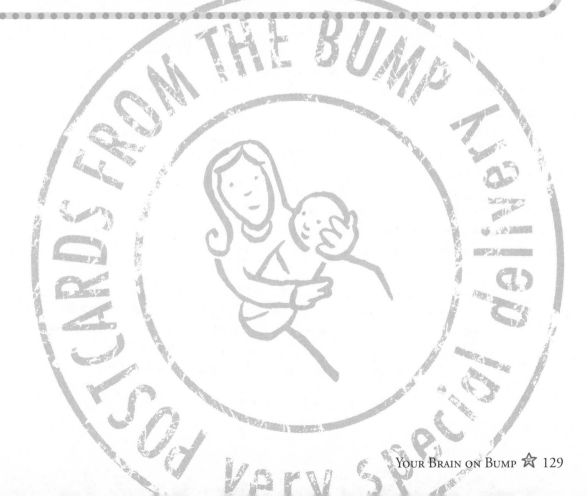

Bump in the Night:
Pregnancy Dreams

"Sweet" may be the last adjective you'd choose to describe your dreams these days. One night you're giving birth to a 12-year-old, while the next you're jumping over puddles filled with tadpoles or swimming with dolphins. With their total suspension of reality and disregard for logic, dreams are the ultimate thrill rides; when you're pregnant, you may have to hold on tighter than usual. During pregnancy, dream-filled REM sleep is disrupted more often than normal, which can make for intense, bizarre dreams. The interrupted sleep patterns, coupled with restlessness, discomfort, and hormonal shifts, can make for a wild nightlife. Dreams—our subconscious way of sorting out emotions, confronting concerns, and addressing conflict—provide fertile ground during life-changing events like pregnancy. Below is a handy chart that might shed a little light on your nighttime adventures.

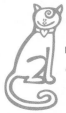

DREAM IMAGES: Animals

POSSIBLE MEANING: Animals can represent qualities you associate with that creature, for example, dogs can stand for loyalty, comfort, and protection; dolphins can signify our spirituality, playfulness, and optimism; frogs represent imminent change, adaptability, and resilience—animal symbology is easy to research in books or online, but the best interpretation is your own take on their significance. Puppies, kittens, chicks, bunnies, and other cuddly, nurture-needing little animals are common images in pregnant women's dreams, and how you relate to the little critters can give insight into your feelings about impending motherhood—comfortable, anticipatory, nervous, and so forth.

DREAM IMAGES: Giving birth to a grown child or having your baby bypass labor and simply "pop" out

POSSIBLE MEANING: Part wishful thinking, part fear of missing out on something, dreams like this are common if you're feeling anxious or inexperienced as a mother. The idea of having an older, more self-sufficient child may seem much less daunting than giving birth to a fragile newborn. And as for skipping labor, that's truly a fantasy for many women!

DREAM IMAGES: Houses, skyscrapers, buildings, factories

POSSIBLE MEANING: Dreaming about renovating or remodeling a house can mirror the physical changes your body is experiencing. Dreaming of places where things are made or spaces that are large in scope correlates to the experience of creating life and anticipating your body/baby's growth. You may feel like a "baby-making factory" or awed by the big changes you feel, see, or are anticipating in your physical shape.

DREAM IMAGES: Water

POSSIBLE MEANING: Water dreams can allude to your amniotic fluid. Dreams of oceans, pools, lakes, and rivers mirror the shifting, amorphous state of your body, as well as your emotions and the mysteries of pregnancy. Near birth, it's common to dream of water in relation to your water breaking—waves, storms, and flowing rivers are common late-term dream images.

Water and its buoyant quality can also symbolize your longing to feel light, weightless, and carefree.

DREAM IMAGES: Flowers, vines, trees

POSSIBLE MEANING: Dreams about nature are often obvious correlations to fertility, creation, and growth. Seeds become plants, bear buds, bloom, bear fruit—their cycles mirror gestation. Often pregnant women dream of things growing wildly, quickly, and out of control, in a lush interpretation of what seems to be happening in our own lives.

DREAM IMAGES: Suitcases, packages, crates

POSSIBLE MEANING: Dreaming about baggage—carrying, moving, or pulling things around—can be a nod to natural fears or trepidation about the responsibilities of parenting and taking care of a baby. It can also represent your desire to get your life and home organized and ready for the baby.

☆ Postcard *to the* Bump ☆

While you were in my belly, I often dreamed of ....
....
....
....

Dream a Little Dream of Me One day out of nowhere, I had severe pains in my stomach and lower back that persisted for more than a week. Work had been stressful, and afraid that I might be nursing an ulcer, I made an appointment with my doctor. The night before, I had one of the most intense dreams I've ever had. I was walking through a forest under a towering canopy of redwoods when I knelt down to pick up a beautiful pinecone. When I stood up, I suddenly had an enormous pregnant belly. I rested my hand on my big bump and kept walking until I came to a clearing that revealed a beautiful bed dressed in blue, luxuriously soft linens. I lay down and like magic there was a perfect little baby lying next to me—and my body was back to normal. That morning I went to the drugstore and got a home pregnancy test—it was positive. My "ulcer" turned out to be a beautiful baby boy. To this day, my son and I have an uncanny sleep connection. I often wake up in the middle of the night, and moments later he'll wake up, too. And most every morning it's the same thing: He wakes up right after I do—I call him my little "sonrise." —Mary

Before you were born I carried you under my heart. From the moment you arrived in this world until the moment I leave it, I will always carry you in my heart.

—*Mandy Harrison*

It Shows I was days into my first pregnancy, and my husband and I had told no one else our exciting news. While out running errands, I stopped by the local bookstore, where an employee asked if I could wait for her as she rang up another customer. When she finished, she came up to me and said, "Can I ask you a personal question?" When I nodded, she asked, "Are you pregnant?" My stunned silence was answer enough. When I asked how she knew she said, "I'm a little psychic, and from the moment you walked in here I could sense the presence of a baby so strongly that it was distracting." She then went on to tell me that the baby she sensed was strong and well and for me not to worry about anything. That encounter was the first of many blessings and fun surprises that that little baby, now aptly named Grace, has bestowed upon me. —Ame

A Mother Hen Told Us... An old wives' tale says that if a woman dreams of a spark, she's seen the soul entering her baby's body.

A mother's heart is the child's classroom. —*Henry Ward Beecher*

We leave it to you, kind reader, to decide whether these are ramblings of precocious toddlers or conditioned memories. Regardless, it's fascinating to consider how pervasive memory can truly be.

"You know, Mimi, it's really hard to be born. I really didn't want to come out. I tried to stay in, but it was very hard so I just came out."

—*Janna, four years old, told to her grandmother*

"Remember how I used to tickle you with my toes when I was in your tummy? I thought that was so funny."

—*Jonathan, six years old, told to his mother*

"Mama, when I was in your belly I was a bird listener. But now that I'm here, I'm a birdwatcher."

—*Grace, five years old*

"I was adopted when I was four weeks old. When I was older, I started having the same dream over and over about green walls, elephants, and giraffes. When I told my mother about it, she told me that when they picked me up from the foster home, the nursery was painted light green and the crib had a mobile with giraffes and elephants on it."

—*Bennett, 12 years old*

Beauty by Bump:
Looking Swell

As a pregnant woman you are both the exception *and* the rule when it comes to beauty. With a little baby tucked under your skin, your beauty suddenly goes far deeper. You embody the age-old truth that it's what's on the inside that matters, and, even better, you get to experience firsthand that beauty is in the eye of the beholder, as evidenced by all the smiles your bump elicits from perfect strangers. The conceptual beauty of pregnancy is easy to grasp—but what's a girl to do when she's feeling a little *too* swell, grieving for her lost ankles, and finding her glow has given way to oily shine? You do what we always do—ask your girlfriends for help. We polled countless chicks and professionals for some tips on bumping up your beauty during pregnancy.

FACE FACTS. With pregnancy hormones raging, you may feel as if your skin has regressed to sophomoric behavior. It's time to put on your "baby face" and tweak your normal skin-care routine. Hydration will fuel that pretty pregnancy glow, so up your water intake and try a new moisturizer based on your skin's new needs. If your skin's oilier, opt for products that are water-based and labeled "noncomedogenic," which means they won't clog pores. Facial blotting paper is a great way to combat shine instead of layering on more powder. Use a broad-spectrum sunscreen every day to reduce discoloration that can occur when hormones trigger the multiplication of pigment cells, often called "pregnancy mask." Now's also a great time to prime for motherhood by simplifying your makeup routine with some multitasking products that will save time and freshen your look. If restless sleep has you packing under-eye bags and dark circles, meet your new best friend—con-

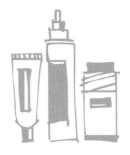
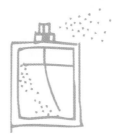

cealer. And never underestimate the power of berry-tinted lip gloss to perk up a preggy.

ACCENTUATE THE POSITIVES. Congratulations—you've won the attention lottery! For better or worse, it seems as if all eyes are on you, so now is the perfect time to flaunt what you've got. If your cups runneth over, dare to share a little peek of that cleavage with sexy necklines and scoop-neck tees. Great legs? Display those pretty stems beneath baby-doll dresses, knee-skimming skirts, and straight-leg pants. Don't go muumuu mama; instead hug your blossoming curves with soft knits and body-skimming styles that celebrate your ripe womanly shape.

LOOK OUT LADY GODIVA. Normally, about 90 percent of our hair is in a "growing state" at the rate of about half an inch per month. The other 10 percent is in a "resting phase" where it hangs on for two or three months before falling out. When you're pregnant, higher estrogen levels can stretch the growing stage; less hair falls out, thus making your hair thicker. It's a great time to wear your hair a little longer, and nothing highlights neck and cheekbones more chicly than a sleek, low ponytail or a playful updo. Use your hair to slenderize a full face by avoiding blunt bangs and cheek-hugging layers.

THIS LITTLE PIGGY WENT "WHEE, WHEE, WHEE" …ALL THE WAY TO THE NAIL SALON. The same hormones that are making everything else grow are also fueling your nails. All that growth positively necessitates manicures and pedicures, so be sure to scratch out some time to pamper your fingers and toes.

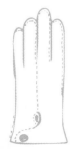
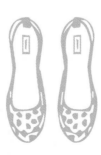
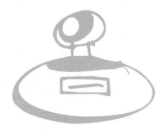

☆ Postcard *to the* Bump ☆

Something that made me feel pretty when I was pregnant was

Beauty is not in the face;
**beauty is a light in
the heart**

—*Kahlil Gibran*

DADDY'S FAUX PREGNANT
Hand Over My Maternity Pants and Nobody Gets Hurt

Most of us hoped for a "modern" man to father our children, but what do you do when Mr. Sensitive suddenly starts acting like a prego-wannabe? Before you scoff at his sudden craving for oranges and demand that he hand over your saltines, be warned that the medical establishment might just back him up. It turns out that more than a quarter of expectant fathers experience Couvade syndrome. Yes, they even came up with a drama-queen name for it. Couvade comes from the French word for "hatched" and means sympathetic pregnancy. Typically "symptoms" begin at the end of *your* first trimester and include mood swings, food cravings, weight gain, toothaches, headaches, itching, nosebleeds, and sometimes even cysts. Although dads managed to get a legitimate label for their suffering (even though it only took until the latter part of this century for the medical establishment to admit that PMS was real), the medical community still hasn't been able to explain the hows or whys yet. Theories on exact causes range from sympathy for their pregnant wives, attention deficit (read: they're just jealous), to a subconscious desire to demonstrate that they really love you (awww).

If your man is a card-carrying Couvade syndrome kinda guy, it might be easier to swallow the medical diagnosis than obsess about how he's trying to steal your thunder. Rest assured, he's probably not going to find a ton of sympathy in the locker room—no matter how modern his buddies are. And thankfully, his little syndrome will be gone as soon as your baby arrives.

As long as you know men are like children, you know everything.

—*Coco Chanel*

A Mother Hen Told Us... Historically, people believed that wet nurses imparted not only nourishment to the babies they fed, but also passed on aspects of their personality—like religious beliefs, intelligence, speech patterns, and emotions—through their breast milk.

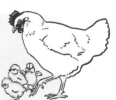

YOUR BRAIN ON BUMP:
Just Call Me Mrs. Smarty Pants

If you swear your brain seems to be shrinking as your bump gets bigger, you're not alone, and you're far from crazy—about 50 percent of pregnant women report feeling more absentminded. But before you bemoan the bump brain drain, consider a University of Richmond–Virginia study asserting that pregnancy actually makes you smarter. Dendrite and glial cells (both affect brain productivity) were found to double in the brains of pregnant mice. As a result of this cellular brain boost, the pregnant mice had a better sense of smell and sight, ran mazes faster, and retained information longer than their bump-free friends. Other studies on pregnancy and memory theorize that a surge of hormones, specifically oxytocin, is responsible for increases in empathy, courage, motivation, and multitasking skills in expectant women as compared to their nonpregnant counterparts.

So how do you explain all those mental lapses at the refrigerator door when you ask, "Now what did I come to get?" Scientists believe the short-term memory loss can be chalked up to less restful sleep, a flood of new information for the brain to process, and sensory overload—things anyone, pregnant or not, would find distracting. As for the smart part, here's the good news—the study concluded that the brain boost was permanent! Being a mom may not give you eyes in the back of your head, but evidently it makes the ones you do have that much keener.

Moms are
the Cheese

Pay close attention to the **little things,** for one day you may look back and realize they **were the big things.**

—*Anonymous*

Stitch in Time Each time I was expecting, I was dead set against finding out the baby's gender. The only thing that kept me going through those difficult last weeks of pregnancy was the anticipation of finding out whether we'd have a boy or a girl. To pass the time, I made crib-sized quilts. I remember scanning the rows of calicos at the fabric store, waiting for just the right gender-neutral colors to jump out at me. As I finished the quilts, each one seemed perfectly suited to a boy or girl. One day, when my children were toddlers playing on the floor with their quilted blankies, my sister asked, "Didn't you make those before Sabrina and Jake were born?" Yes, I had. "But you didn't find out the sex when you went for your ultrasound?" "That's right." I had wanted to be surprised. "I don't believe you," she said. Looking at the blankies, I could understand my sister's disbelief: My daughter's "gender-neutral" quilt was a purple floral with pink and blue accents. My son's? Blue and white! I may not have found out the genders of my babies, but something inside me knew. —*Shannon*

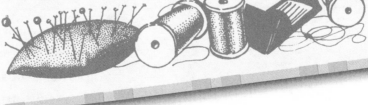

No one knows what ultimately triggers labor. The due date, unless you're having a scheduled Caesarean, is a guesstimate at best and one of the few genuine unexplained mysteries of pregnancy. In this chapter, we explore ways in which you can embrace motherhood and share tips on getting through the transition, including surviving those first few months with baby. We give you ideas for getting the most out of your baby showers, find ways to get you fed, and share some wonderful stories about the emotional welcome of a baby. We hope the information here will not only ease your fears but embolden you to face motherhood on your very own terms.

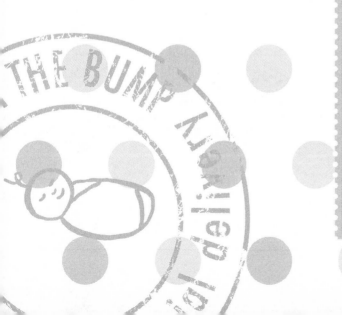

POSTCARDS FROM THE BUMP

HAVING A BABY DOESN'T TURN
YOUR LIFE UPSIDE DOWN AS MUCH
AS IT TURNS YOUR HEART
INSIDE OUT.
—*Ame and Emily*

5   5

DEAR MOM, things are going swimmingly well in here. It's a little like Vegas—hard to tell day from night but I'm so cozy I don't really care. Can you believe I just perfected my triple flip? Did'ya feel it? I can't believe I got three full rotations in this tight space—just wait 'til I get on the outside. I'm gon... ...adruple roll. It's gonna be sweet! LOVE YOU, the Bump... ...know you can't feel me or hear me yet but I am so here... ...say "hello," soon. Forever Your Girl or Boy, the BUMP... ...must have been some kin... ...person who lau... Oh, and I loved... think I heard s... of that. Yours truly, the... ming voice and that last tu... whatever you played in th... standing. But that classical...

CHAPTER FIVE • 5

Ready to Rock
Shake, Rattle, and Roll

DEAR MOM, I think I need a bigger womb. Sorry about all the kicking, but a baby's gotta stretch the little legs once in a while. I swear, either this place is shrinking, or I'm getting HUGE! And the sounds—whoa! When that fire truck came by last night I thought I was going to jump right out of your skin! Give Dad my love and tell him to back up to the belly, and I'll give him a few little kicks. Your Growing BUMP Sparkling

Double or Nothing: A Cautionary Tale

During my second pregnancy my descent into mommy mania began simply enough—I was pushed.

I blame my decline on the countless mothers who warned me how hard it was to go from one child to two. "Like going from zero to sixty," one mom yelled to me over her shoulder as she dashed to retrieve her oldest from scaling a tree while her toddler raided her purse, gleefully popping Tic Tacs into her tiny mouth. It was after the ninety-ninth person informed me that the birth of my second was sure to bring us to our knees that my insubordination began to bubble. A little attitudinal pushback started simmering inside, and I decided that not only were they fear mongers, but I'd also show them just how wrong they were. I hung my mutinous mommy hat on the flawed logic that they just refused to acknowledge that having one baby was backbreaking, too. I had endured too many sleepless nights with our daughter to buy into the "two-is-harder-than-one" argument. This would not be my first time at the all-night rodeo.

As my "mommytude" grew, so did my bump, and our second child, a boy, was born healthy and perfect with a wonderful tendency to *sleep*. It's a little-known secret that an infant who sleeps too well from the get-go can be hazardous to your health—especially if you're already wielding a supermom ax to grind. I've come to view sleep deprivation as a twisted form of self-preservation, because when you're too tired to get dressed and all you want to do is assume the fetal position on the couch, any efforts to impress or champion a cause fly out the window.

Instead, during my maternity leave I took on as much as I could—hosting playdates for my daughter, stenciling the nursery, making home-made chicken potpie. A trip to the beach? Sure, I'll pack the sandwiches. In-laws for lunch? No problem, I'll devil some eggs. But as the weeks rolled by, my manic spirit began to head south. I was unraveling, and there was nothing pretty about the precarious piles of laundry hiding in my closets or the bags forming under my eyes.

"Honey, why don't you take a nap today?" my husband suggested as I buzzed around. I refused, of course, citing the statistical impossibility of getting two children to sleep at the exact same time. Plus our vacation was approaching. I was too delusional to realize that you actually should *rest up* in anticipation of a family vacation with two young children. In my stubborn craze to outwit, outplay, and outlast, I did the opposite: I insisted on doing all the shopping for the five families (with ten children) for our Cape Cod vacation and planned a Costco expedition for the day before our departure.

Things got off to a promising start—the little guy slept in the baby seat while my daughter sat in the cart fiddling with a new toy I had brilliantly brought along. We were rocking and rolling as I cruised every aisle, consulting my list to make sure all 20 individual food preferences were satisfied. When I finished, the cart was so full that I could just make out a tuft of my daughter's hair peeking out from behind the boxes. With the baby still asleep I rolled the cart down a cement ramp into the blazing-hot parking lot. I paused in the bright sunlight to imagine the reception I'd receive as the

When my kids become **wild and unruly,** I use a nice, safe playpen. When they're finished, **I climb out.**

—*Erma Bombeck*

other moms gushed with gratitude over my shopping coup. "How did you manage?" one would marvel, or perhaps, "Two kids sure haven't slowed you down!"

I was imagining it all when my daughter stood up in the cart.

"Sit down. It's not safe," I hissed. She had a two-year-old's mastery of "No!" and as I went to grab her, the cart lurched forward . . . and she slo-moed into a backward dive over the front. She hit the cement with a sickening sound.

Stricken and terrified, I cradled her as she wailed and was relieved to discover that she'd miraculously suffered nothing more than a skinned elbow. As I hugged her, I looked up to see the fully loaded cart, with a still-sleeping infant, careening down the ramp like the iconic baby carriage in *Battleship Potemkin*. I started screaming—the window-shattering, eardrum-splintering scream that only a truly terrified mother can make—and watched as another shopper deftly stopped the cart in its tracks.

Fighting tears, I held my daughter's hand and pushed the cart to our car. Once the kids were buckled in, I called my husband, who listened patiently, the way someone patronizes a crazy person. As I went over the details, I noticed that my right shoe was missing—it hadn't even registered that I was walking on hot pavement with one bare foot. For a split second I considered retrieving the

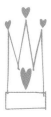

I am **convinced** that if given just the right outfit and **a proper tiara**, I could save the world.

—*Anonymous*

lost flip-flop, but the prospect of baring my sole again kept me riveted to the seat. I wondered if I could call an ambulance and be sedated while they drove us all home.

You can get just about anything at Costco, and fortunately I found a huge helping of exactly what I needed that day—perspective. The incident, as scary as it was, jarred me to my senses, and I abandoned my Super Mom ambitions on the spot. I realized that even though parenting, regardless of family size, isn't always considered the hardest job in the world, it is indisputably the most important, and when you take on too much the fundamental things—like the safety of your children—can be tough to ensure. Motherhood is a competition only in regard to achieving your personal best, and while it's devoid of year-end bonuses, corner offices, or gold medals, the smiles, giggles, and hugs that punctuate our days can't be beat.

Martyr Smarter: Remove Thyself from the Mommy Masochism Poster

Martyrdom is so five centuries ago, and no one looks pretty rendered in stained glass anyway. So toss aside the guilt and give yourself a big break. Take this simple quiz to evaluate your risk of mommy masochism.

In the first three months after your baby was born, have you ever been tempted to:

1. Locate your skinny jeans?

2. Adopt a puppy so your baby has a best friend to grow up with?

3. Enroll in a 6 a.m. pilates class?

4. Entertain a single, party-girl college girlfriend for the weekend?

5. Bake a raspberry pie from scratch, replete with a lattice-work top?

6. Wash your windows?

7. Host the neighborhood playgroup?

8. Have sex?

If you answered yes to any one of these questions, you have one foot on the slippery slope to the mommy masochism abyss. Begin your retreat by immediately taking the following steps away from the precipice of this backbreaking, rampant disease:

Although prepared for martyrdom,
I prefer that it be postponed.

—*Winston Churchill*

1. Buy a new nonmaternity outfit that fits and flatters (if you can't get out of your house, order multiple sizes online and mail back what doesn't fit).

2. Take a daily shower and blow-dry your hair at least twice a week.

3. Get a haircut.

4. Find some household help (be it man, woman, or child, enlist aid with taking out the trash and folding all those tiny baby onesies and bibs).

5. Exercise, meditate, or just get out and take a walk for at least 30 minutes a few times a week—alone. Anything done while pushing a stroller, sporting a baby in a sling, or bouncing one on your hip does not count.

6. Schedule a night out on the calendar to look forward to (even if it's six weeks away).

Remember, life now isn't about raising the bar, it's about raising your hand when you need help, and raising a family. Don't forget yourself along the way.

A Mother Hen Told Us... Mothers should act like babies—nap when she naps, have water or tea when he nurses or takes a bottle, play when she's in the mood, take a bath together, and surrender to the slower pace that little feet require.

The **most important thing** she'd learned over the years was that there was no way to be a perfect mother and a **million ways to be a good one.**

—*Jill Churchill*

Bump Up the Volume My youngest bump was in a big hurry to get here, so together we spent many an hour hooked up to beeping machinery and noisy hospital monitors. Maddy's premature debut required a two-week hospital stay where she charmed the nurses with her easygoing nature and great sleeping habits. An atypical preemie, she would snooze for four-hour stints amid the wailing and fussing of her tiny new friends. We were ecstatic when we finally got to take her home, and since her two-year-old sister still wasn't sleeping through the night, the thought of a "sleep-trained" newborn made us feel even more blessed. But something happened when we crossed our threshold . . . to our dismay she began to cry and bellow practically nonstop.

We rocked, we paced, we drove her around in the car, but she would not be soothed until one afternoon I walked into the game room where our family was watching a football game. The cacophony of a blaring TV, people yelling, and kids laughing startled me, but before I could rush out, something miraculous happened—I felt Maddy relax in my arms. That's when it clicked. Maddy liked noise. She couldn't sleep because it was too quiet. I recalled how my little bump had always slept through our preterm labor hospital stints—ironically lulled by the beeping and buzzing. As we searched for the perfect noise, she loudly vetoed sound machines, music, and static until we found the sweet sound of success by taking the batteries out of the smoke alarm in her room. The intermittent beeping was music to her ears. She logged eight hours that first night, and I didn't sleep a wink for anxiously checking on her. Maddy's now five, but to this day you will find her asleep on the living room floor in front of a blaring TV or dozing at the holiday table amid a crowd of loud relatives. The kid can sleep through anything . . . except silence! —Jessica

Gone are the formal tea-sipping, daisy-strewn, yellow-tinted affairs of our mothers. Today's baby showers can be anything you want them to be—as long as you celebrate your bump and serve the very practical purpose of gearing you up for the arrival of your baby. Be sure to get the most out of your showers by focusing on a few key things.

SET THE TONE. Soon enough you'll be caught up in the whirlwind of newborn care, so don't feel guilty about commandeering the baby showers for a little "you" time. While your family or friends will, with luck, plan a thoughtful shower, a little direction and some positive suggestions from you will do wonders. You don't have to go control freak on everyone and orchestrate every detail, but if you'd prefer chintz to seersucker, mocktails to iced teas, or buffet to sit-down, let your hosts know. Don't be afraid to suggest a few easy themes or stylish "jumping-off points" for your shower hostess. Favorite foods, color cravings, and personal de-tails will all make your shower positively sunny. Look to the "Shower Brainstorm" section (p. 151) for some shower inspiration.

REGISTERING 101. The best rule of thumb for baby registry is to keep things simple. If you're a first-time mom, try and consult an experienced mom (or ask her to come along with you to register) and check out a book on baby products for de-scriptions and reviews. Don't make your baby-gift registry so big that it overwhelms you and your guests, and though you're talking about your bundle of joy here, don't go off your rocker. Do you really need a fancy stroller that rivals the price of your first car, or three different types of slings? Think long term and register for clothing in a variety of sizes and consider items that you'll need as baby grows. Note a simple nursery theme or outline a color scheme to inspire your guests' gift selections, and be sure to have your reg-istry details and information done in time to include in the shower invitations.

Shower Brainstorm: Stylish Baby Shower Themes

"Once Upon a Time"

Stock your little bookshelves with a children's book–themed baby shower where guests are asked to give their favorite childhood book or select one from a registry at a local bookstore. Décor can be as simple as dressing up hardcover books with dust jackets made from pastel or patterned papers and stacking them up to display fresh flowers and candles on. Print quotes from classic children's books on pastel cardstock and hang them festively, banner-style, from ribbons. Handmade bookmarks make sweet parting favors. Thank your hostess with a gift certificate to her favorite bookstore, a customized embosser, book plates, or a book-lover's journal.

"Happy Nests"

Have a true hen and chick party with a sweet little setting that pays homage to our feathered friends. For a centerpiece, cluster craft-store nests filled with speckled eggs, rosebuds tucked in water tubes, or even pairs of tiny shoes. Inexpensive wooden birdhouses painted in solid colors give a chic chick vibe, and don't forget to ruffle some feathers by scattering pastel-tinted feathers whimsically on tabletops or displaying them in bowls and vases. Have guests use paint pens to write notes on one of the birdhouses for a sweet take on the guest book that can be added to baby's nursery. Individually boxed truffles in little nests of shredded paper make great gifts for your peeps. Show your appreciation to the little bird who put it all together with a set of luxury bird's-egg soaps, a diminutive birdbath for her garden, or a blown-glass hummingbird feeder.

Singing in the Rain. Give a classic theme an update with décor that incorporates centerpieces made of trays of wheatgrass studded with vibrant gerbera daisies, flower-filled vases tucked into children's rain boots, watering cans, and colorful Chinese paper parasols suspended from the ceiling with ribbons. Seed packets of your favorite flower tied up with tulle are the perfect way to make a splash with your guests. Your hostess will bloom when you thank her with her favorite scented candle and bubble-bath duo or a fetching new umbrella.

THE GREEN BEAN. Organic, nontoxic, recycled, and eco-friendly gifts are the focus of this "love your mother" fest. It's a great opportunity for your mom friends to share gently used baby clothing that can pull double duty as décor when you display them on a ribbon clothesline. Make centerpieces of potted plants that can be added to the garden, or landscape and repurpose baby-food jars filled with wildflowers and tied with raffia. Thank guests for coming with a canvas shopping tote tied with pretty ribbon. Thank your green party girl

What the bump wants, the bump gets!

Nest Cookies

2 C all purpose flour
1 T baking powder
¼ tsp salt
¾ C butter
1 C granulated sugar
¾ tsp vanilla extract
2 C coconut, flaked
1 8-ounce package cream cheese
1 12-ounce bag candy-coated chocolate almond candies

Preheat oven to 325 degrees. Coat cookie sheets with nonstick spray.

Sift together the flour, baking powder, and salt; set aside.

In a medium bowl, cream butter, cream cheese, sugar, and vanilla until smooth. Gradually stir in sifted dry ingredients.

Roll dough into 1 ½-inch balls, then roll the balls in the coconut. Place balls on cookie sheet two inches apart and gently press your thumb into each to form an indentation. Sprinkle each with a little more coconut.

Bake for 12 minutes, then remove from the oven and press three candies into each nest. Return to the oven and bake for another four minutes, until golden brown.

Let cool before transferring to a cake stand for serving.

Makes 24 cookies.

A baby will **make love stronger,** days shorter, nights longer, bankrolls smaller, homes happier, the **past forgotten,** and the future worth living.

—Anonymous

with an organic cotton tee and a gourmet basket filled with fair-trade delectables.

SHOWERED WITH ADVICE. Along with an invitation, send friends and family a small scrapbook page with a request to share their tips for happy parenting, or a favorite childhood tradition, or to impart their particular brand of life wisdom. Host a casual gathering to collect all those sage sentiments, and let your friends know how much you appreciate their support. Decorate with baby photos of your guests (gathered in advance) and play a game of who can come up with the best "yearbook caption" for each photo. Customized fortune cookies give everyone something sweet to savor as they leave. Thank your hostess with a photo album embossed with her initials.

MAMA SAID SEW. Invite guests to decorate a square of fabric to be transformed into an instant heirloom quilt for your baby. Encourage mediums from traditional embroidery and patches to more contemporary embellishments like paint pens and iron-ons—make sure everyone signs his or her name to their square. Host a series of evening quilting bees to put your quilt together, or prevail upon a professional to whip it into shape. Decorate your shower with a clothesline where everyone can display their fabric squares. Play a game and ask everyone to guess whose square is whose. Favor your guests with some soothing hand cream and thank your hostess with a gift certificate to her favorite craft supply store.

THE MOM-AND-POP SHOWER. Perhaps Daddy really wants to get in on the shower game, or maybe you just can't imagine celebrating your baby without him at your side. Co-ed showers can be a real hoot—as there's nothing like a little testosterone to ramp things up a bit. Forgo frilly and adopt a retro theme. Be sure to have something filling for the guys to graze on—chili and cornbread or a substantial pasta dish will keep everyone happy. Serve popcorn in carnival bags and hand out bubblegum cigars and Sugar Daddys to departing guests. Play "Spin the Baby Bottle" and create a pool to guess name, birth weight, or baby's birth date. Thank your hostess with a gift certificate to a cool diner or favorite restaurant.

THE GIRLFRIEND "BABY" POWER SHOWER. Even if you're expecting a boy, there's nothing like a dose of girl time to prepare you for impending mommyhood. Get the gals in on the fun with activities such as Henna tattooing, pink and blue pedicures for all (especially those who can't reach their toes), and mini-facials. Have your girlfriends make a "Meet Your New Mommy!" book all about you and your family for the new baby. Serve delicate finger foods, petits fours, white chocolate fondue, pink lemonade, and nonalcoholic Jell-o shots as a tribute to the good old days. Give your hostess a haute accessory from your favorite boutique as a thank-you.

What the bump wants, the bump gets!

Raspberry Swirl White Chocolate Fondue

For the raspberry sauce:
1 C fresh raspberries
⅛ C kirsch or framboise (raspberry liqueur)
½ C confectioners' sugar
2 T fresh lemon juice
Puree all the ingredients in a food processor and remove and strain the sauce to remove the seeds; refrigerate.
12-ounce bag white chocolate chips
⅔ C heavy cream
2 T brown sugar
1 T corn syrup
2 T butter
2 T light cream

Melt the white chocolate in a fondue pot with heavy cream.

Place over medium heat and stir constantly until chocolate has melted and is smooth and creamy. Place sugar, corn syrup, and butter in a small pan and heat gently until blended. Remove from the heat and stir in light cream. Pour sugar, corn syrup, and butter into the white chocolate.

Pour raspberry sauce on top of the fondue in a swirl, then serve immediately.

Serve with pineapple, pears, strawberries, melon, and Italian biscotti cookies for dipping.

Serves 8–10

Getting by with a ~~Little~~ Lot of Help from My Friends

It all began the moment we brought our baby home from the hospital. Exhausted, I only got as far as the couch, where I plunked down to nurse her. Too tired to even reach for the remote, I looked around the room. Something was terribly wrong. Things were out of place—or, more precisely, things were *in* place. Our CDs were back in their cases; my collection of pregnancy magazines had been stacked neatly on our coffee table; and the dust bunnies were gone from the corners where they were usually held captive by spider webs.

"Honey . . . did YOU clean the house?" I asked, knowing that my husband hadn't had a second here alone since I went into labor. He smiled, sat down beside me, and said, "Your friends borrowed a key while we were in the hospital." I did the only thing an overly hormonal, totally worn-out new mom could do: I wept uncontrollably at their kindness and foresight. It was a wonderful feeling to finally see the floor of my closet and have a freshly made bed.

But it didn't stop there. Next came the food deliveries—five-layer Mexican casserole, beef stew, pasta salad, and peanut-butter brownies—all homemade and delicious. Like magic, a tasty meal arrived every day right in time for dinner. As soon as I was a little more mobile and up to answering the phone, the offers of help came pouring in. "Would you like me to come over and hold the baby while you sleep or take a shower?" my friend Alice asked. A few hours later she cradled my daughter while I took a long, luxurious shower.

Really? I was speechless. I had never been in a position to have help so generously offered, and while it felt wonderful, I can't say it was entirely comfortable.

And then the presents began to arrive—a gift certificate for a massage and facial, with a babysitter to boot! A handmade baby quilt, fruit baskets, flowers—everything came with the same condition: Accept the gift only if you don't write a thank-you note!

How could our friends and family be so prescient and considerate?

Chalk it up to hormones, but very soon after the gifts started streaming in, I began to feel overwhelmed with anxiety, preoccupied with thoughts of how I was ever going to thank everyone. I was up to my eyeballs in "friendship debt," and the reciprocation I felt it demanded had me teetering on the edge. As the favors and acts of kindness continued to roll in, so did the sinking feeling that I could never repay everyone for all their efforts. Like a shopaholic receiving unsolicited credit cards, I began to think I was being setup for failure. What if I got so delinquent, overdue, and bankrupt that all my friends were repossessed?

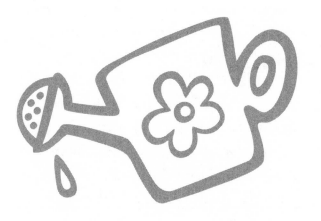

Learn to write your hurts in the sand and carve your blessings in stone.

—*Proverb*

When my friend Jamie came to the door with another delicious meal—this time macaroni salad—I thought I would fall to my knees in despair.

"I tried to make the same recipe that you made for us, but I don't think it's quite as good," she said.

"I made YOU this recipe?" I stammered, as I admired the colorful homemade macaroni salad. "Yes, just after Elle and I got home from the hospital. It was so delicious. I lived on it for a week." She smiled.

I thought back, and even in my postpartum haze I did vaguely recall making some macaroni salad and doubling the batch. It was so little trouble that I barely remembered it. But that was two years ago—and Jamie still remembered!

Then it hit me—you can't measure gratitude as you measure other things. The burden of a task on the giver does not correlate with how much it relieves the recipient—the impact is not measured by effort, but by the spirit of the people involved in the exchange. So focused was I on repaying my debts, I didn't realize that the mere enjoyment of their generosity could be payment enough. I humbly realized that none of my friends were keeping score—and neither should I.

As my eyes welled up with grateful tears, Jamie hugged me tightly, saying, "Hey, it's just pasta. It was easy."

I simply said, "Thank you. It just means so much to us."

I blamed my hormones for the rush of emotions, and we laughed as I went inside to savor every bite of that deeply satisfying and soul-nourishing macaroni salad.

Praise the bridge that carried you over.

—*George Colman*

What the bump wants, the bump gets!

Mama-Macaroni Salad

1 pound small macaroni elbows
½ C olive oil plus 1 teaspoon
2 T red wine vinegar
juice of 1½ lemons
¼ tsp dried mint
¼ tsp dried oregano
3 peppers, 1 each red/yellow/green, diced
1 brunch broccoli, chopped
1 cucumber cut in ½ lengthwise and chopped
8 oz Greek olives
1 small red onion
1 pint cherry tomatoes, halved
8 oz pasteurized sheep's milk feta cheese

2 cloves minced garlic
Salt and pepper to taste

Cook macaroni according to package directions. Rinse macaroni under cold water, drain, turn into a bowl, and toss with 1 tsp olive oil. Steam the broccoli until tender, then let it cool. Slice the red onion and immediately put slices into a bowl of ice water for about five minutes. Mix the remaining olive oil, vinegar, lemon juice, mint, oregano, and garlic into the macaroni. Add the remaining ingredients, toss well, and add salt and pepper to taste. Serves 8–10.

The Five Friends Every New Mama Needs

Months into the game, I had finally learned the valuable lesson of why people try really hard to make babies look cute:

1) They are perfect for deflecting attention away from yourself.

2) If they look good, they can make you look better.

3) A mom with a dirty, disheveled baby looks like a crazy person.

-Beth Lisick

SISTER FROM **ANOTHER MISTER.** When you need someone who will feel your fury over your husband's insistence on keeping up his "golf game," or your own aggravation over your baby's refusal to nap, she's your gal. No matter what the prenatal experience, this empathetic buddy understands your pain and offers up her shoulder to cry on. She won't look at you askance when you complain about your bizarre postpartum symptoms—in fact, she thinks she had that, too, and it's as awful as you think it is. She's the one you go running to after another brutally sleepless night or after your mother-in-law comes to town. Though not usually solution-oriented, she has big ears and an even bigger heart, and the minute you tear up she'll well right up with you in tender solidarity.

MAMA MADONNA. This mama has clocked a lot of time in the sandbox and is generous with her BTDT (been-there-done-that) advice. She's the one who can quickly discern the difference between a hungry cry and a sleepy one, when a boo-boo needs more than a kiss, and she can spot promising "babysitter meat" a mile away. She successfully walks that fine line between annoying know-it-all and wise woman, as she knows when to listen and when to dispense.

HONEST BABE. She's the straight shooter who will tell you when your super-sized nipples are visible and when your child should go home because those puffy eyes look contagious. If you need an honest answer about whether junior's cradle cap has crossed the line from invisible to revolting, she's the one to sidle up to. Although she isn't someone you can handle spending every day with, especially if you're feeling fragile, a little dose of her honesty every once in a while can be just what you need.

IMAMA. This gadget guru has or has tried every cool baby-related item ever introduced into the infant industrial complex. Need the latest in nightlight soothing technology? She can point you in the right direction. Hoping to find a diaper robo-genie that magically empties itself? She knows where you can get it—at half price! As indispensable as a fresh diaper and a generous supply of wet wipes, iMama constantly prowls parenting

> # I really learned it all from mothers.
>
> —*Dr. Benjamin Spock*

websites and baby boutiques to give you the latest for your precious bundle.

CALAMITY JANE. If Homeland Security (and by "home," we mean your very own address) is top on your list, you'll want this mama to keep you up to date on the latest in toxins, viruses, and any other potential hazards that might threaten your baby. Overcautious to the point of complete mania, she sure comes in handy when it comes to installing car seats, and she'll be the first to send you e-alerts about the latest product recalls. Good at fueling your paranoia—and creating it, too—she has read the latest studies on everything from plastic nipples to lead paint.

Re-Building Blocks: Mommy Edition

As much as you get out of pregnancy—cleavage, a bigger heart, and, best of all, a sweet baby—we'd be big fat liars if we pretended the whole process didn't suck a whole lot out of you as well. Sleep is what most of us moms focus on getting, but replenishing yourself nutritionally is important not only for your physical well-being but also for your mental and emotional health. In Chapter One, we outlined some food recommendations for when you're pregnant (Baby Building Blocks p. 43), but we'd like to point out how important your *post*-delivery diet is, since pregnancy depletes your body of a host of vitamins, minerals, and fatty acids. While we encourage you to avoid junk food, refined sugars, white bread, and empty calories, depriving your body is like forgetting to bring your baby's car seat to the hospital—it's irresponsible and dangerous. Your body needs essential fatty acids, calcium, iron, and a too-long-to-name list of other vitamins and minerals. But before we work you into a postpartum tizzy, take

heart that eating well doesn't require intense recipes or tedious food prep. Here are some healthy, easy-to-access foods to include in your diet that will aid both body and mind.

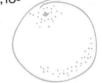

- **BROCCOLI** is rich in fiber, calcium, folate, antioxidants, and vitamin C.
- **FORTIFIED BREAKFAST CEREALS** are chock full of vitamin B and folate.
- **CHEESE** delivers satisfying taste plus calcium and protein.
- **OMEGA-3 FORTIFIED EGGS** deliver protein, healthy omega-3s, the antioxidant vitamin E, and docosahexaenoic acid (or DHA), which has been shown to boost serotonin levels.
- **BANANAS** are easy snacks for those on the go, and they also pack a punch of energy-boosting potassium.
- **ORANGES** are the classic source for vitamin C.
- **NUTS AND NUT BUTTERS** a delicious source of protein, fiber, and essential fatty acids.
- **WHOLE-GRAIN BREADS** provide an easy serving of fiber, folate, and vitamin B.

Ancestors 101: Decorating with Family Pictures

Give your baby a homecoming replete with adoring fans, thanks to a family photo gallery in her nursery. It may be a while before she can focus clearly, but being surrounded by loving faces will serve as a "welcoming committee" for the newest little bud on the family tree. Research shows that while newborns can't clearly see faces, they do respond to them more enthusiastically than to images of inanimate objects. So dust off your favorite shot of Uncle Charlie and pull Great-Grandma out of the attic—it's time to decorate the nursery.

EXCITE WITH BLACK AND WHITE. Babies see black and white better than color, so convert your photos for maximum baby interest. This will also unify photos from different eras so that Grandpa Bob's navy uniform won't look so odd next to childhood shots of Daddy wearing tie-dyed tee shirts.

FOCUS ON THE FRAMES. A hodgepodge of inexpensive frames or flea-market finds instantly jive if you paint them all the same color. Scour your closets for old frames and unify them with a crisp

> Family faces are magic mirrors. Looking at people who belong to us, we see the past, present, and future.
>
> —*Gail Lumet Buckley*

coat of white, black, metallic, or accent color from your nursery. Don't be totally square—inject ovals and offbeat shapes, too. Black-and-white photos framed in bright colors like hot pink, apple green, or periwinkle blue can give a fresh and sophisticated vibe to a collection of art and photos.

MAKE THE MATTES MEANINGFUL. For an eclectic look or sentimental touch, have family members write notes on the mattes for their photos. "I've loved you from the moment I got the good news of you—Love always, Grandma Karen," or "You're gonna rock! Your new best friend—Cousin Sam," will be sweet stories for your little

The family. We were a strange little band of characters trudging through life sharing diseases and toothpaste, coveting one another's desserts, hiding shampoo, borrowing money, locking each other out of our rooms, inflicting pain and **kissing to heal it in the same instant,** loving, laughing, defending, and trying to figure out the **common thread that bound us all together.**

—*Erma Bombeck*

one to grow up with. Photocopy colored fabrics that you're using in the nursery to surround photos, or make collages on the mattes with postcards, letters, or pages from your favorite children's books.

MIX IT UP. For maximum impact, group family photos together, and don't be afraid to inject a piece of artwork here and there for pop. Add a framed photo of baby's first ultrasound; a masterpiece by an older sibling; a shadowbox with your silver spoon, a scrap of Daddy's blankie, or other family "treasures"; and don't forget to anchor it all with a shot of you and your big, beautiful bump.

FAMILY TREE CHIC. For whimsy, hang a real tree branch horizontally on the wall and cluster frames around it for "family tree" funk. Hot-glue some silk cherry blossoms or velvet leaves to the branches for cottage chic, spray-paint the branch a bright high-gloss color for contemporary punch, or tuck in a few nests for garden-inspired pizzazz.

A Spoonful of Sugar: Sweet Escape

If you're having a hard time avoiding the "sweeter" aisles in the supermarket, it could be more than just your stomach propelling you there. Research indicates that when we eat sugar and sweets, receptors in our mouths trigger our brains to release natural morphine-like chemicals called endogenous opiates that give us a sense of pleasure and well-being. Studies have also shown that the taste of a sweet substance helps to reduce crying and fussiness in babies. What's more, sweets are purported to promote baby's alertness and the development of hand-to-mouth coordination. Both the fats and sugars in breast milk are extremely beneficial to infants, so if you're nursing, feed and hydrate yourself generously. But before you beat a path to the ice-cream shop, remember that too much refined sugar isn't good for you or baby. Naturally sweet satisfaction can be found at the fruit stand or by making yourself a nutritious smoothie (p. 105) instead.

What the bump wants, the bump gets!

Velvety Lemon Squares

For the crust:
2 C sifted flour
½ C confectioner's sugar
¼ tsp salt
1 C butter (chilled)

For the lemon mixture:
4 eggs
2 C granulated sugar
⅓ C fresh lemon juice
1 ½ tsp grated lemon rind
¼ C flour
1 tsp baking powder
Confectioner's sugar for dusting

Preheat over to 350 degrees.

In medium to large bowl sift together 2 cups flour, ½ cup confectioner's sugar, and salt.

With pastry blender or two knives cut the butter into flour mixture until mixture clings together and resembles coarse meal. Press mixture evenly into a 9x13 pan. Bake crust for 20 minutes or until lightly browned. Cool 10–15 minutes.

In a large bowl beat eggs and slowly add granulated sugar. Blend in lemon juice and rind into egg mixture. Sift together ¼ cup flour and baking powder and add into egg mixture and blend. Spread lemon mixture evenly over baked slightly cool crust and return to oven for 25 minutes.

Cool on pan or rack and sprinkle with confectioner's sugar and cut into squares.

Makes about four dozen bars.°

Since ancients times, birthstones have been given to babies and their parents as tokens of good luck. Aside from the sentiment and tradition of wearing a meaningful piece of jewelry, birthstones, much like astrological signs, signify certain personality traits for the individual whose birth month they represent. Have a little fun considering what your baby's birthstone might reveal about that little gem in your belly.

JANUARY • GARNET shines with constancy, faithfulness and even temperedness.

FEBRUARY • AMETHYST represents genuineness, honesty, and sincerity.

MARCH • AQUAMARINE wearers are brave, audacious and courageous.

APRIL • DIAMONDS are symbolic of purity, innocence, and naivete.

MAY • EMERALD is the gem of success—green like money, it heralds prosperity.

JUNE • PEARL is the stone of longevity, good health, and perseverance.

JULY • RUBY with its rosy color is the stone of happiness, love and contentment.

AUGUST • PERIDOT people are passionate, loving and have wonderful relationships.

SEPTEMBER • SAPPHIRE babies are wise, insightful and discerning.

OCTOBER • OPAL gemstones are full of fire and light signifying hope and optimism for their wearers.

NOVEMBER • TOPAZ is warm in color as well as spirit for it signifies friendship and unity.

DECEMBER • TURQUOISE signifies wisdom, honor and wealth.

Sip-and-See: Baby's Day Out

Everyone wants to meet the precious little baby that the bump has become, but entertaining guests should be the absolute last thing on your to-do list. When you feel up to it, usually about two to four weeks after the baby's born, enlist a friend or family member to host a "sip-and-see" at her home where people can do just that—pop in for a quick refreshment and a brief visit with mama and baby. Sip-and-sees are short—no more than two hours—and can be open-house casual. That way when friends call and ask, "When can we come see the baby?" you can make sure to tell them to the put the "sip-and-see" on their calendars.

Forget the Silver Spoon When Grace was born via C-section there was this quiet moment just before they pulled her out—then everyone in surgery erupted in laughter—"What? What is it?" I asked, "What's so funny?" Was my baby that funny-looking? My doctor said, "It's a Baby Grace, and she was born with her foot in her mouth." She was breech with a foot basically beside each ear, and she had taken to sucking her toes while in utero! Thankfully she did not carry on that habit, but she is the most flexible creature I've ever seen. We call her our little contortionist. And she has a real knack for expressing herself that we call "foot in mouth" syndrome. —Ame

A Mother Hen Told Us... Your shower hostess may be throwing you the mother of all parties, but there's no reason to stress when it comes to expressing your appreciation. Show up the day of the event with a simple gift—a plant, guest towels, a book, stationery, gift certificate to download music—and write her a sweet note after the party. See "Shower Brainstorms," p. 151, for some thematic inspiration.

Baby announcements are the absolute sweetest correspondence to ever grace a mailbox. While e-mails are great for letting friends and family know your little bump has landed, there's something extra-special about sharing the precious news via post. Planning a design, choosing a stamp, and addressing envelopes are a great way to pass the snail's pace of time in those final weeks waiting for baby. Etiquette suggests mailing your announcements before your baby turns one month old. Here are some inspired ideas for sharing your good news.

POSTCARD OF THE BUMP. Print or handwrite baby's stats on pastel postcard paper. Have U.S. postal stamps made featuring your baby's picture at www.photostamp.com. Without removing stamps from their backing, cut them out of the sheets and affix a stamp to each postcard using removable double-stick tape so friends and family can keep or use the stamps to mail a little note of their own. Mail your cards in pink or blue envelopes.

SWEETIE PIE RECIPE. Affix your baby's photo to a recipe card and include a fun headline like "Cutie Pie," "Recipe for Happiness," "Our Pumpkin Is Here," or "Cupcake" and write recipe-inspired details: "7 pounds, 8 ounces of sugar, 20 inches long, ready to eat up on March 2, 2009."

HEIR MAIL. Paste a photo of your baby onto a piece of craft-colored cardstock and, using a "Received" stamp set to his birth date, stamp the card. Using a typewriter-inspired font, print file-folder labels with his name and weight and add them to the card for a nostalgic announcement.

Mail the cards using classic "airmail" envelopes.

SWEETPEA. Print baby's photo and stats on printable sticker project paper (available at office supply stores) and affix stickers to seed packets of baby's birth flower so recipients can add your little blossom to their own gardens. For bulbs, nestle a cellophane-wrapped bulb in a small box, include your announcement and planting instructions, wrap in brown paper, and mail for an extraordinary blooming announcement.

OVER THE MOON (AND STARS). Research the constellation for your baby's zodiac sign and print it on the front of a folding card. Inside, under the headline "Our Little Star," share a photo of his shining little face and all the stellar details. Mail using metallic envelopes.

T-TOTALLY CUTE. Using your computer and iron-on transfer paper, create a onesie that has your baby's name, birth date, and weight and photograph her wearing it. Or you can scan a photo of your baby wearing a solid-colored onesie and add the words to the shirt. Either way, your little one will make quite the style statement!

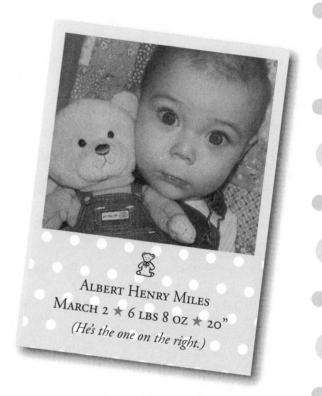

ALBERT HENRY MILES
MARCH 2 ★ 6 LBS 8 OZ ★ 20"
(He's the one on the right.)

Birth announcements harken back to the Victorian era, when personal calling cards ceremoniously reported people's visits and invitations. Formally, they were small cards simply stating the baby's full name and birth date, which were placed on top of a larger card with the parents' names.

Little Buds: Birth Month Flowers

January • Carnation

February • Iris

March • Daffodil

April • Daisy

May • Lily

June • Rose

July • Delphinium

August • Gladiola

September • Aster

October • Marigold

November • Chrysanthemum

December • Poinsettia

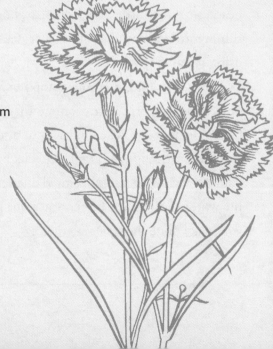

Are You Ready? Baby Knows Best

With all we know through modern prenatal medicine about the health, size, gender, genes, and even appearance of our babies before they're born, it's surprising that science still hasn't been able to pinpoint exactly what triggers birth. There are endless wives' tales about what causes labor—everything from tea and sex to pedicures and overexcitement. For years, many doctors believed that something in the mother's body somehow caused labor to begin, but recent studies on animals have scientists pointing their fingers at the baby as instigators.

These studies suggest that birth is triggered by the release of hormones from the baby's brain. So if things work similarly in humans, one theory suggests that baby's glands release a hormone that begins the birthing process by triggering a cascade of hormones that come together to stimulate contractions in the mother. However it happens chemically, the fact that scientists believe that baby's brain integrates all the information needed to tell whether it's ready to be born is pretty extraordinary. That's a lot of responsibility for someone so little to shoulder!

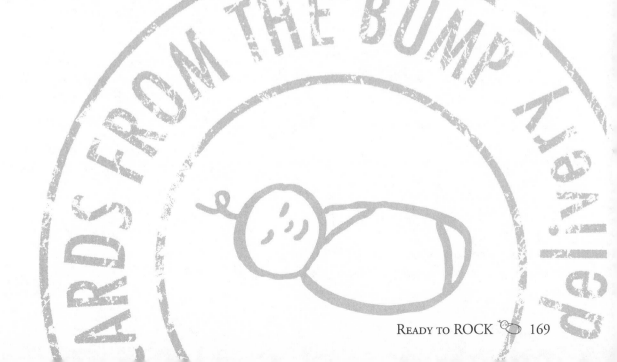

Since You Asked . . . Suggestions for Wannabe Do-Gooders!

Most people have a pretty good idea of what they can do to help out a new mom, but there are always those well-intentioned types who really want to help but need a little direction. That's where these recipes come in. As soon as that sweet neighbor or your great Aunt Ida asks "What can I do to help you?" hand her one of these recipes or ask her to help you stock up on items from p. XX Rebuilding Mama. If you feel a tad guilty, tell her that you're just following doctor's orders.

PLEASE NOTE: If they can't cook or shop, potential do-gooders fall into the baby-holding category, so ask them to hold your little bundle of joy while you shower or nap. If they can't do that, you really need to send them on their merry way until your baby can walk.

Little Monkey Muffins

These muffins are delicious and great for a quick bite any time throughout the day and night.

4 ripe bananas, mashed, plus another ripe banana, thinly sliced for garnish
1 C brown sugar, packed
1 omega-3 egg
½ C canola oil
1 C all-purpose flour
1 C whole-wheat flour
1 tsp baking powder
1 tsp baking soda
½ tsp salt
½ C sour cream
1 T vanilla extract
½ C chopped pecans

Preheat oven to 350 degrees. Spray muffin tins with nonstick vegetable oil. Mash bananas with a fork; stir in brown sugar, egg, and oil. Using a handheld mixer, beat on medium until smooth.

With mixer on low, gradually mix in the flour, baking powder, baking soda, and salt until smooth. Mix in sour cream and vanilla extract.

Fill muffin tins about ¾ full. Sprinkle each muffin with chopped pecans and top with a slice of banana.

Bake 25 minutes until a toothpick inserted into the muffin comes out clean.

Makes 18 muffins.

Salmon and Swiss Puff Pastry Quiche

This nutritious quiche variation is easy and full of omega-3 oils and vitamins.

2 sheets frozen puff pastry (one 17-ounce package), thawed
1 C salmon lox, sliced into ½-inch squares
2 C Swiss cheese, grated
1 C asparagus, sliced into small pieces
3 large omega-3 eggs
1 T fresh rosemary, chopped
½ tsp ground black pepper
½ tsp salt
¼ tsp ground nutmeg
1 C low-fat sour cream

Preheat oven to 400 degrees.

Bring a pot of water to a boil and drop in asparagus for 30 seconds. Remove asparagus and drain well in colander.

Unfold one puff pastry sheet into each of two pie pans. Top with salmon, cheese, and asparagus, leaving edges of pastry border uncovered.

Whisk eggs, rosemary, pepper, salt, and nutmeg in bowl. Slowly add sour cream, stirring well. Spoon egg mixture over toppings on each pastry. Bake until pastries are puffed and golden and toppings are set, about 25 minutes. Variation: if you don't like salmon, substitute ham, turkey, or sautéed mushrooms.

Serves 6 to 8.

Pasta Salad with Chicken, Tomatoes, and Corn

This is another wonderful, eat-anytime recipe. The chicken, fresh tomatoes, and corn make it a powerful snack or side to go along with dinner.

5 T olive oil
5 T red wine vinegar
½ C fresh basil, chopped
2 large garlic cloves, chopped
1½ C fresh corn kernels (cut from three ears) or frozen and thawed
1¼ pounds plum tomatoes, chopped
2 chicken breasts, cooked and shredded
8 ounces penne pasta, freshly cooked
½ C grated Parmesan cheese

Whisk four tablespoons of the oil, the vinegar, and basil in large bowl to blend.

Heat remaining oil in large heavy skillet over medium heat; add corn and garlic, sauté three minutes, then add to dressing in bowl.

Add tomatoes, pasta, chicken, and cheese to bowl; toss to blend. Season salad with salt and pepper.

Onesies of a Kind: Tees for Tots

Before you know it, your bump will be running around exhibiting her own unique fashion sense. Until that day, revel in one of motherhood's sweetest joys—projecting your own sense of style onto a helpless little protégé. Make a big statement with your tiny one by creating personalized onesies and tee shirts with printable iron-on transfer paper (available at craft or office supply stores) and blank apparel.

> Before you were conceived I **wanted you.** Before you were born I loved you. Before you were here an hour I would die for you. This is the miracle of **Mother's Love.**
>
> —*Maureen Hawkins*

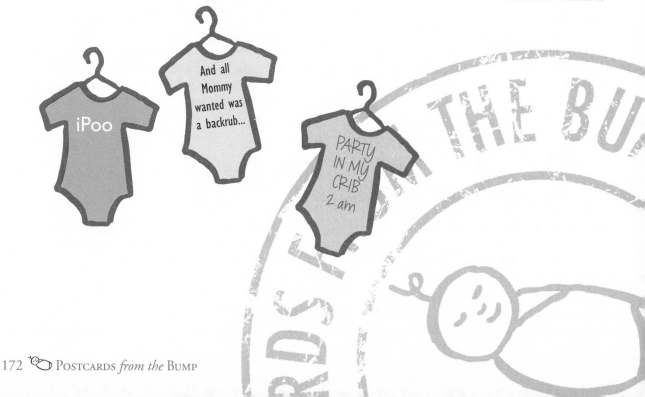

iPoo

And all Mommy wanted was a backrub...

PARTY IN MY CRIB 2 am

Born to Be

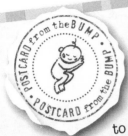

Justin's labor was 26 hours long. He was stubborn and would not budge. Similarly he has always proven to be very head-strong, strong-minded, and a bit pessimistic. His first reaction to anything is "no." When my second, Halle, was born, however, she was a little freight train. I barely made it to the hospital, no IV, no epidural, no doctor present. Consequently she is my "yes" girl and is very social and eager to try new things. Number three, Anna, was a typical labor—not too fast or too slow. She has a balanced temperament that is between the other two! —Wendy

A Mother Hen Told Us...

Monday's child is fair of face;
Tuesday's child is full of grace;
Wednesday's child will fear no woe;
Thursday's child has far to go;
Friday's child is loving and giving;
Saturday's child works hard for a living.
But the child that is born on the Sabbath day
is fair and wise, good and gay.

Ame & Emily ❧ Who are these chicks?

Ame Mahler Beanland and Emily Miles Terry are the *New York Times* bestselling authors of *Nesting: It's a Chick Thing®* and the bestselling *It's a Chick Thing®: Celebrating the Wild Side of Women's Friendship.* Ame and Emily are columnists for Disney's www.FamilyFun.com and www.family.com where they regularly write on parenting and family lifestyle topics. Ame plays house in the Dallas area with her husband and two children. Emily nests in the Boston area with her husband and three children. Visit them online at www.itsachickthing.com

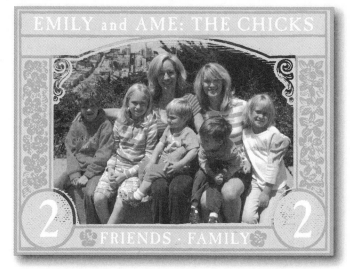

That's us with our little "eggs."

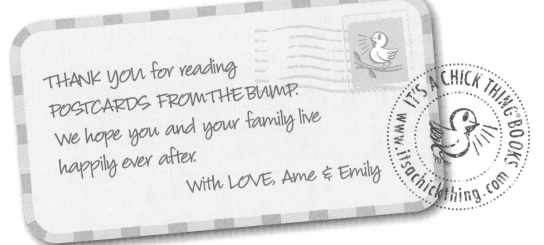

THANK you for reading POSTCARDS FROM THE BUMP. We hope you and your family live happily ever after.

With LOVE, Ame & Emily

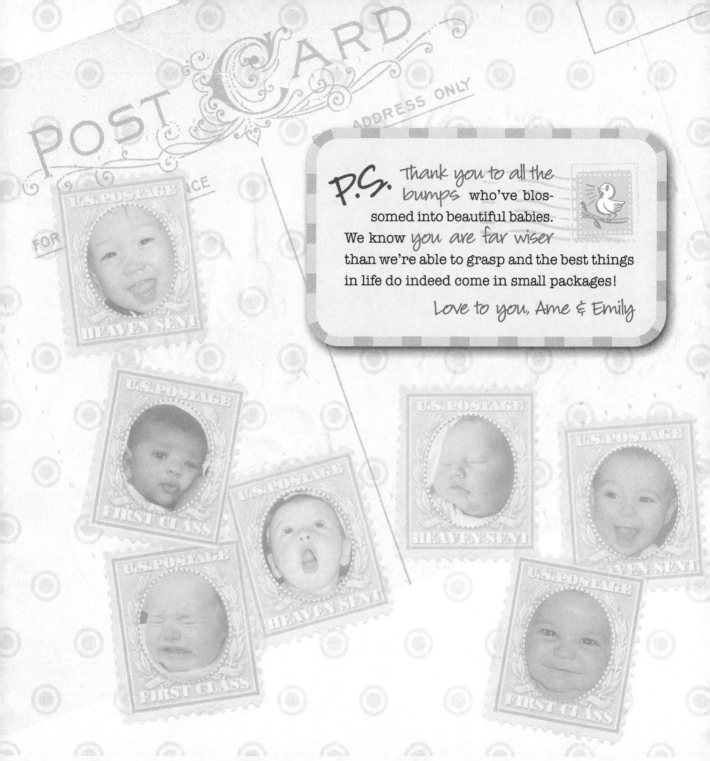

POST CARD

FOR ~~CORRESPONDENCE~~

ADDRESS ONLY

P.S. thank you to all the bumps who've blossomed into beautiful babies. We know *you are far wiser* than we're able to grasp and the best things in life do indeed come in small packages!

Love to you, Ame & Emily

U.S. POSTAGE — HEAVEN SENT

U.S. POSTAGE — FIRST CLASS

U.S. POSTAGE — HEAVEN SENT

U.S. POSTAGE — FIRST CLASS

U.S. POSTAGE — HEAVEN SENT

U.S. POSTAGE — HEAVEN SENT

U.S. POSTAGE — FIRST CLASS

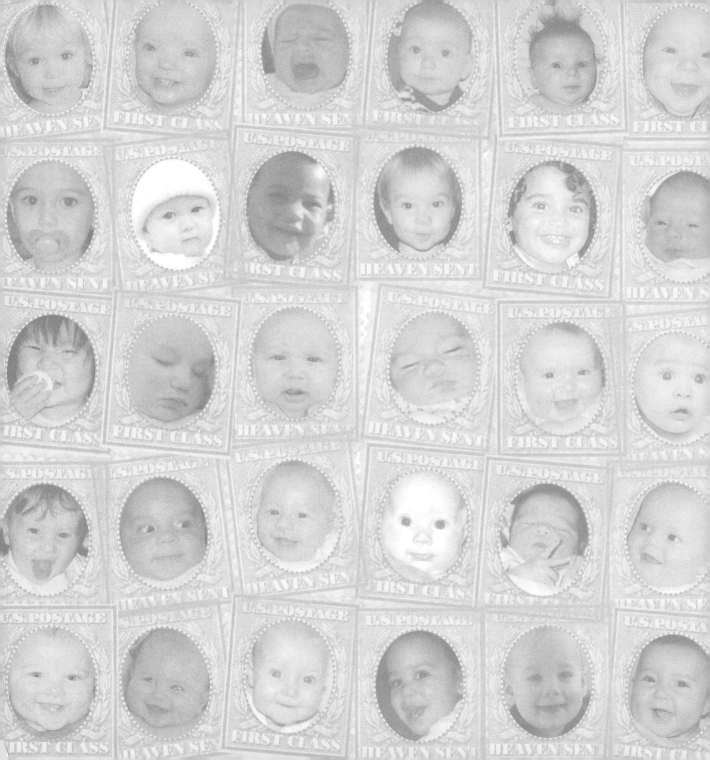

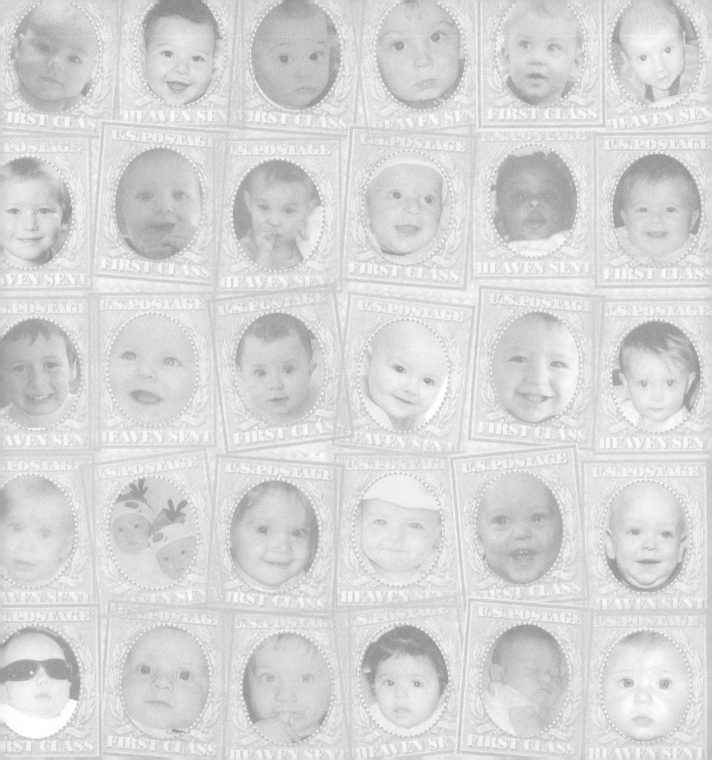

Acknowledgements

It takes a village to write a bump book! To all the chicks who helped us nurture this book into existence, we express our deepest gratitude for your fertile and generous spirits. We especially want to thank our agent, Jenny Bent, for her support and enthusiasm for all our ideas—you turn them into books. To our editor Wendy Francis, at DaCapo Books, thank you for adopting our "baby" and loving it like your own. We owe our lives to our mothers, Karen Miles and Mary Mahler, who keep us fired up and never fail us. And to our fathers, Tom and Albert—you are forever in our hearts.

To Ame's big sister Kathy and Emily's grandparents, Emily and Hans, whose inspirational and gentle support help keep us on track.

To our "roosters" Dave and Peter, thank you for all your support, for being our biggest fans, for holding down the nest while we swap stories and most of all, for helping us hatch our greatest works—Julia, Henry, Miles, Grace and Luke.

Thank you to all our contributors, muses, and collaborators whose input is always invaluable:

Janna Absher	Lisa Bryant	Sue Dolezal
Susie Albert	Kristen Bush	Jill Bauer Dunne
Rachna Balakrishna	Angie Buster	Rosalba Fuentes Echavarria
Wendy Barner	Celia Carrasco	Beth Edelsten
Kristen Barney	Veronica Carter	Marlene Eldred
Tammy Barney	Rose Coronado	Mary Eng
Patricia Barille	Abby Cox	Jody Fidler
Karen Bauer	D'Lissa Cunningham	Colleen Fisher
Marietta Beanland	Cindy Cutlip	Kristine Flinn
Jessica Begley	Andrea Dillard	Ellen Groustra
Kellie Blumberg	Laura Dietrick	Caitlyn Hagerty

Joan Hansen

Laura Hansen

Eve Harris

Melissa Holaday

Lisa Hodgins

Uno Immanivong

Molly Intfen

Kristin Jain

Susan Janosky

Paula Joyce

Karen Kastigar

Renata Knight

Tammy Knight

Shannon Lane

Margie Lapanja

Anne Large

Stacey Larsen

Donna Lord

Theresa Mahler

Shelby Martindale

Aimee Miles

Karen McCarthy

Susan McMurry

Nancy Milla

Jennifer Mitchell

Ashley Moore

Carrie Morris

Andria Mraz

Suzanne Newell

Andrea Noe

Diana Nygren

Ellen Oberle

Carolyn Otto

Catherine Patience

Bridget Patton

Linda Phelan

Jill Pollack

Alicia Powell

Justina Quick Radcliff

Christy Reppetto

Rhonda Revels

Talisha Revels

Sheryl Rifas

Shannon Riggs

Amy Rinzler

Nancy Roberts

Janna Robertson

Kathy Robertson

Lisa Rodriquez

Heather Rose

Leslie Rossman

Susie Ruth

Mary Jane Ryan

Cisca Schreefel

Susan Senator

Lynette Shirk

Thea Singer

Kim Sloan

Elisabeth Socolow

Jayne Sullivan

Ruth Sullivan

Melissa Harty-Swaleh

Renita Tankersley

Tracey Teare

Beth Teitell

Sherelle Thompson

Renee Turcott

Maria Luisa Victoria

Karen Vifian

Micqualyn Waldie

Kellie Wright

Sources

Prenatal Memory

A. J. DeCasper. "Recurring Auditory Experience in the 28-to 34-Week-Old Fetus." *Infant Behavior and Development*.

A. J. DeCasper and W. P. Fifer. *Of Human Bonding: Newborns Prefer Their Mother's Voices. Science*, June 6, 1980.

N. L. Gonzalez-Gonzalez et al. *Persistence of Fetal Memory into Neonatal Life*. (Acta Obstetricia et Gynecologica Scandinavica 2006).

Thomas Verny. *The Secret Life of the Unborn Child* (Summit Books, 1982).

Prenatal Hearing and Maternal Voice Recognition

A. J. DeCasper and W. P. Fifer. *Of Human Bonding: Newborns Prefer Their Mother's Voices. Science*, June 6, 1980.

W. P. Fifer. *The Role of Mother's Voice in the Organization of Brain Function in Newborn*. (Acta Paediatricia Suppl., June 1994).

D. Querlu. "Reaction of the Newborn Infant Less Than 2 Hours After Birth to the Maternal Voice." *Journal de Gynecologie Obstetrique et Bioglogie de La Reproduction*, 1984.

Astrology

Rae Orion. *Astrology For Dummies* (For Dummies, 2d ed., 2007).

Joanna Woolfolk. *The Only Astrology Book You'll Ever Need* (Taylor Trade Publishing, 2008).

Prenatal Smell

Lise Eliot. *What's Going on in There? How the Brain and Mind Develop in the First Five Years of Life.* (Bantam, 1999).

Taste and Food Preference

Lise Eliot. *What's Going on in There? How the Brain and Mind Develop in the First Five Years of Life.* (Bantam, 1999).

Amniotic Fluid Flavoring and Taste in the Fetus

J. A. Mennella. "Prenatal and Postnatal Flavor Learning by Human Infants." *Pediatrics*, June 2001.

Fetal Movement

Bornstein et al. "What Does Fetal Movement Predict About Behavior During the First Two Years of Life?" *Developmental Psychobiology* vol. 40, 4: 358–371. Published Online, April 17 2002.

Glade B. Curtis, MD, MPH and Judith Schuler, MS, *Your Pregnancy Week by Week* (Perseus, 6th ed., 2008).

Couvade Syndrome in Males

H. Klein. "Couvade Syndrome: Male Counterpart to Pregnancy." *International Journal of Psychiatry in Medicine*, vol. 21, 1991.

Susan Magee. *The Pregnancy Countdown Book* (Quirk Books, 2006).

Prenatal Hearing

C. Brezinka et al. *The Fetus and Noise* (Gynako Beburtshilfliche Rundsch, 1997).

Glade B. Curtis, MD, MPH and Judith Schuler, MS, *Your Pregnancy Week by Week.* (Perseus, 6th ed., 2008).

Dietary Needs of Fetus and Mother

Associated Press. "Eat Fish, Beat Postpartum Blues." May 2003.

Jim Bourre. "Dietary Omega-3 Fatty Acids for Women." *Biomed Pharmacother*, Feb–April, 2007.

Glade B. Curtis, MD, MPH and Judith Schuler, MS, *Your Pregnancy Week by Week.* (Perseus, 6th ed., 2008).

I. Hosli et al. "Role of Omega 3-Fatty Acids and Multivitamins in Gestation." *Journal of Perinatal Medicine*, 2007.

Zita West. *Babycare Before Birth: The Prenatal Program That Gives Your Baby the Best Start in Life* (Dorling Kindersley, 2006).

Morning Sickness

Miriam Erick. Managing Morning Sickness: A Survival Guide for Pregnant Women (Bull Publishing, 2004).

Fetal Movement

Glade B. Curtis, MD, MPH and Judith Schuler, MS, *Your Pregnancy Week by Week*. (Perseus, 6th ed., 2008).

A. Kurjak. "Behavioral Pattern Continuity from Prenatal to Postnatal Life." *Journal of Perinatal Medicine*, 2004.

Hormones

T. Baumgartner. "Oxytocin Shapes the Neural Circuitry of Trust and Trust Adaptations in Humans." *Neuron,* May 22, 2005.

BBC News. "Scientists Create 'Trust Potion.'" June 2005.

Maternal Emotions and Impact on Fetus

B. R. Can den Bergh et al. "The Effect of (Induced) Maternal Emotions on Fetal Behaviour: A Controlled Study." *Early Human Development*, April 19, 1989.

D. C. Geary., "Sex Differences in Behavioral and Hormonal Response to Social Threat." *Psychol. Rev.,* 2002.

S. E. Taylor et al. "Biobehavioral Responses to Stress in Females: Tend and Befriend, Not Fight or Flight." *Psychol. Rev.*, October 2002.

Things to Make and Do Index

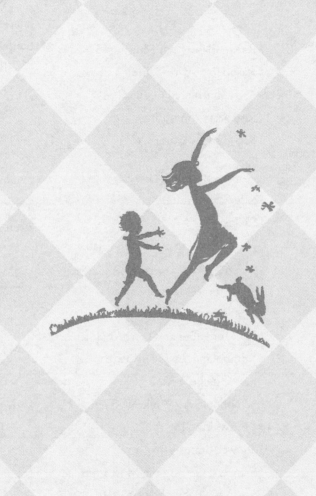

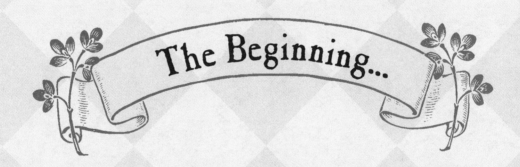

The Beginning...